The Hospital Laboratory

MODERN CONCEPTS OF MANAGEMENT,
OPERATIONS, AND FINANCE

The Hospital Laboratory

MODERN CONCEPTS OF MANAGEMENT, OPERATIONS, AND FINANCE

R. M. SHUFFSTALL, M.D.

Riverview Hospital Association
Wisconsin Rapids, Wisconsin

BRECHARR HEMMAPLARDH, Ph.D., M.B.A.

Abbott Laboratories
Abbott Park
North Chicago, Illinois

*with **44** illustrations including **19** forms with four color coding*

The C. V. Mosby Company

ST. LOUIS · TORONTO · LONDON   1979

To those with whom we have
shared the experience
of providing laboratory services

The C. V. Mosby Company
11830 Westline Industrial Drive, St. Louis, Missouri 63141

Library of Congress Cataloging in Publication Data

Shuffstall, R   M   1924-
  The hospital laboratory.

  Includes index.
  1. Medical laboratories—Management.   2. Medical
laboratories—Finance.   I. Hemmaplardh, Brecharr,
1942-   joint author.   II. Title.
RB36.S58   658'.91'616075   78-11877
ISBN 0-8016-4620-0

TS/CB/B   9   8   7   6   5   4   3   2   1   02/A/217

PREFACE

The hospital laboratory has evolved from a service unit to a business entity. Unfortunately, this change has been brought about by circumstances more than by intentions. Gone are the days when its sole responsibility was to respond to the needs of physicians. The traditional role of producing laboratory data to aid in the diagnosis of diseases and to follow the progress of therapy has been greatly expanded. It is no longer sufficient to be technically competent and scientifically innovative.

Today the laboratory is more visible. It is forced to imagine itself as a business without sacrificing or compromising its traditional role. It must frequently justify its financial needs and account for its performance. Random pricing is under attack. The pooling of risks necessitates accountability to third parties.

Change is brought about by several social and political movements. Hospitals are no longer charitable institutions. Financial resources are limited while costs relentlessly increase. The rising expectation of health care as a right can no longer be ignored and has prompted the call for a more comprehensive system of delivery from the public sector. In addition, malpractice suits have generated much discontent from physicians.

The evolution of the modern hospital laboratory has

produced a chasm between technical competence and scientific innovation on the one hand and inadequate management skills on the other. This book is written to help bridge this chasm by presenting an understanding of the processes essential to cope with the laboratory's changing role. The presentation is divided into four parts. Part one will outline the historical development of the hospital laboratory leading to the current trends and alluding to future prospects. Part two deals with the fundamental concepts for planning, organizing, and directing the hospital laboratory. Part three elaborates on a series of basic operating concepts. A range of greatly needed modern financial concepts and techniques is discussed in Part four.

The most pressing issue in any organization is communication. Much effort was spent in designing and perfecting an inexpensive, simple, and effective request/report form system. These unique forms and accompanying instructions for their use are included in Chapter 5, Communication.

Finally, the highlight of all the controversies to come is anticipated in Chapter 13. It touches on the well-known practice of arbitrary pricing. For those in despair, we offer a systematic model that we hope will signal the beginning of some logic in the important matter of pricing laboratory protocols.

R. M. Shuffstall
Brecharr Hemmaplardh

CONTENTS

PART THREE

MODERN OPERATING CONCEPTS

7 Research and method development, 86

8 Quality control, 91

9 The care of equipment and laboratory safety, 111

PART ONE

Introduction

1

GROWTH AND DEVELOPMENT OF THE HOSPITAL LABORATORY

The American health care industry has an excellent growth record. According to the Department of Health, Education and Welfare, by 1980 health care delivery will contribute 9.7 percent of the gross national product, up from the current 8.6 percent. With a national health insurance program, the same health care cost could consume anywhere from 10.5 to 11.7 percent of the GNP by 1980, depending upon which program is legislated.

The Social Security Bulletin, July 1978, reports that the nation spent a total of $162.6 billion for health care during fiscal year 1977—from July 1, 1976 through June 30, 1977. This figure represents an average of $737 per person, an increase of 12 percent over the estimated $145.1 billion spent in 1976 (Table 1-1).

Health care expenditures continue to increase at a greater rate than the GNP. Fiscal year 1977 spending levels for health care were 12 percent higher than those for the previous 12 months, while the GNP increased by 10.2 percent in the same period. Thus, the health care share of the GNP has grown from 8.7 percent for the year ending September 1976 to 8.8 percent in fiscal year 1977 (Fig. 1-1).

Since much of the health care provided in the United States is obtained in hospitals, the largest category of spending in 1977 ($65.6 billion, or 40 percent of the total)

TABLE 1-1

Aggregate and per capita national health expenditures, by source of funds, and percent of gross national product, selected fiscal years 1929-1977

Fiscal year (ending June)	Gross national product (in billions)	Health expenditures								
		Total			Private			Public		
		Amount (in millions)	Per capita	Percent of GNP	Amount (in millions)	Per capita	Percent of total	Amount (in millions)	Per capita	Percent of total
1929	$ 101.3	$ 3,589	$ 29.16	3.5	$ 3,112	$ 25.28	86.7	$ 477	$ 3.88	13.3
1935	68.9	2,846	22.04	4.1	2,303	17.84	80.9	543	4.21	19.1
1940	95.4	3,883	28.98	4.1	3,101	23.14	79.9	782	5.84	20.1
1950	264.8	12,027	78.35	4.5	8,962	58.38	74.5	3,065	19.97	25.5
1955	381.0	17,330	103.76	4.5	12,909	77.29	74.5	4,421	26.47	25.5
1960	498.3	25,856	141.63	5.2	19,461	106.60	75.3	6,395	35.03	24.7
1965	658.0	38,892	197.75	5.9	29,357	149.27	75.5	9,535	48.48	24.5
1966	722.4	42,109	211.56	5.8	31,279	157.15	74.3	10,830	54.41	25.7
1967	773.5	47,879	237.93	6.2	32,026	159.15	66.9	15,853	78.78	33.1
1968	830.2	53,765	264.37	6.5	33,725	165.83	62.7	20,040	98.54	37.3
1969	904.2	60,617	295.20	6.7	37,680	183.50	62.2	22,937	111.70	37.8
1970	960.2	69,201	333.57	7.2	43,810	211.18	63.3	25,391	122.39	36.7
1971	1,019.8	77,162	368.25	7.6	48,387	230.92	62.7	28,775	137.32	37.3
1972	1,111.8	89,687	409.71	7.8	53,214	251.50	61.4	33,473	158.20	38.6
1973	1,238.6	95,383	447.31	7.7	58,715	275.35	61.6	36,668	171.96	38.4
1974[1]	1,361.2	106,321	495.01	7.8	64,809	301.74	61.0	41,512	193.27	39.0
1975[1]	1,454.5	122,716	571.21	8.5	71,348	329.42	57.7	52,368	241.79	42.3
1976[1]	1,625.4	141,013	645.76	8.7	80,831	370.16	57.3	60,182	275.60	42.7
1977[2]	1,838.0	162,627	736.92	8.8	94,185	426.78	57.9	68,442	310.13	42.1

[1]Revised estimates.
[2]New federal fiscal year.

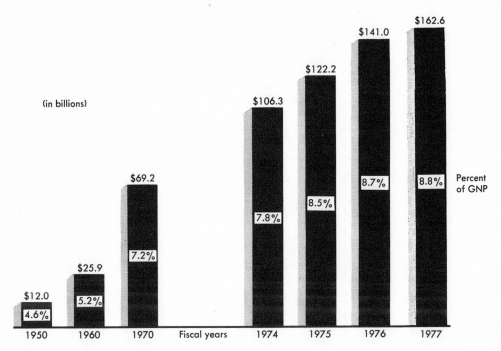

FIG. 1-1
National health expenditures and percent of gross national product, selected fiscal years 1950-1977.

was for hospital care (see Table 1-2). The American Hospital Association estimates that approximately 11 percent ($7.2 billion for 1977) of the total hospital revenues are attributed to payments for laboratory services.

What are the factors accounting for such phenomenal growth? Few astute observers would offer any single reason. In the case of the hospital laboratory, it seems clear the explanation lies with a variety of scientific, technical, professional, political, and of late, medicolegal developments.

Any inquiry into these forces would certainly acknowledge the major role of the researchers and the abilities of the equipment and product manufacturers who efficiently

5

TABLE 1-2
National health expenditure, by type of expenditure and source of funds, fiscal years 1974-1977 (in millions)

Type of expenditure	Total	Source of funds					
		Private			Public		
		Total	Con-sumers	Other[1]	Total	Federal	State and local
		1977[2]					
Total	$162,627	$94,185	$87,807	$6,378	$68,442	$46,563	$21,879
Health services and supplies	153,887	91,294	87,807	3,487	62,594	42,542	20,051
Personal health care	142,586	85,465	82,574	2,891	57,121	39,823	17,299
Hospital care	65,627	29,427	27,887	1,540	36,199	25,715	10,484
Physicians' services	32,184	24,360	24,318	42	7,824	5,808	2,016
Dentists' services	10,020	9,520	9,520	0	500	310	190
Other professional services	3,212	2,288	2,175	113	924	683	241
Drugs and drug sundries	12,516	11,373	11,373	0	1,143	614	529
Eyeglasses and appliances	2,086	1,956	1,956	0	130	66	64
Nursing-home care	12,618	5,434	5,343	91	7,184	4,204	2,980
Other health services	4,322	1,105	0	1,105	3,217	2,424	793
Expenses for prepayment and administration	7,572	5,829	5,233	596	1,743	1,430	313
Government public health activities	3,729	—	—	—	3,729	1,289	2,440
Research and medical-facilities construction	8,739	2,891	—	2,891	5,848	4,020	1,828
Research[3]	3,684	284	—	284	3,400	3,139	261
Construction	5,055	2,607	—	2,607	2,448	881	1,567
		1976					
Total	$145,102	$83,560	$77,470	$6,090	$61,542	$41,648	$19,894
Health services and supplies	136,368	80,726	77,470	3,256	55,642	37,669	17,973
Personal health care	126,217	75,740	73,043	2,698	50,477	34,990	15,488
Hospital care	57,497	25,470	24,013	1,457	32,028	22,538	9,490

Physicians' services	28,504	21,628	21,588	40	6,876	5,059	1,817
Dentists' services	8,987	8,519	8,519	0	468	290	177
Other professional services	2,849	2,136	2,029	107	713	508	204
Drugs and drug sundries	11,472	10,396	10,396	0	1,076	585	491
Eyeglasses and appliances	1,986	1,864	1,864	0	121	65	56
Nursing-home care	10,834	4,718	4,633	86	6,115	3,615	2,500
Other health services	4,088	1,007	0	1,007	3,081	2,329	752
Expenses for prepayment and administration	6,628	4,986	4,427	558	1,643	1,378	265
Government public health activities	3,522	—	—	—	3,522	1,301	2,221
Research and medical-facilities construction	8,734	2,834	—	2,834	5,900	3,979	1,921
Research³	3,623	274	—	274	3,348	3,096	252
Construction	5,111	2,559	—	2,559	2,551	883	1,669
Total	**$127,719**	**$73,238**	**$67,375**	**$5,862**	**$54,481**	**$35,899**	**$18,583**

1975

Health services and supplies	119,771	70,300	67,375	2,924	49,472	32,589	16,883
Personal health care	110,665	65,630	63,211	2,419	45,035	30,290	14,745
Hospital care	49,973	21,348	20,035	1,313	28,626	19,534	9,092
Physicians' services	24,553	18,382	18,346	36	6,171	4,427	1,745
Dentists' services	8,034	7,587	7,587	0	447	270	177
Other professional services	2,463	1,913	1,817	97	550	378	172
Drugs and drug sundries	10,582	9,609	9,609	0	973	510	463
Eyeglasses and appliances	1,822	1,710	1,710	0	112	63	49
Nursing-home care	9,620	4,185	4,107	77	5,436	3,100	2,336
Other health services	3,616	896	0	896	2,720	2,009	711
Expenses for prepayment and administration	6,016	4,670	4,164	506	1,346	1,108	238
Government public health activities	3,091	—	—	—	3,091	1,191	1,900
Research and medical-facilities construction	7,947	2,938	—	2,938	5,009	3,310	1,700
Research³	3,132	278	—	278	2,854	2,612	242
Construction	4,815	2,660	—	2,660	2,155	697	1,458

¹Includes spending by philanthropic organizations and for industrial in-plant health services.

²Preliminary estimates.

³Research and development expenditures of drug companies and other manufacturers and providers of medical equipment and suppliers excluded from "research expenditures" but included in the expenditure class in which the product falls.

⁴Revised estimates.

Continued

7

TABLE 1-2

National health expenditure, by type of expenditure and source of funds, fiscal years 1974-1977 (in millions)—cont'd

Type of expenditure	Total	Private			Public		
		Total	*Consumers*	*Other[1]*	*Total*	*Federal*	*State and local*
				1974[4]			
Total	$106,321	$64,809	$59,836	$4,973	$41,512	$27,499	$14,013
Health services and supplies	99,330	61,584	59,836	1,748	37,746	24,928	12,818
Personal health care	91,315	57,259	56,039	1,220	34,056	22,974	11,082
Hospital care	41,020	19,594	19,081	513	21,426	14,534	6,893
Physicians' services	19,742	15,083	15,069	14	4,659	3,363	1,296
Dentists' services	6,870	6,544	6,544	—	326	211	115
Other professional services	1,929	1,497	1,459	38	432	284	148
Drugs and drug sundries	9,416	8,684	8,684	—	732	400	331
Eyeglasses and appliances	1,674	1,583	1,583	—	91	50	41
Nursing-home care	7,450	3,649	3,619	30	3,801	2,277	1,524
Other health services	3,214	625	—	625	2,589	1,855	734
Expenses for prepayment and administration	5,483	4,325	3,797	528	1,158	995	164
Government public health activities	2,531	—	—	—	2,531	959	1,572
Research and medical-facilities construction	6,991	3,225	—	3,225	3,766	2,571	1,195
Research[3]	2,527	227	—	227	2,300	2,078	222
Construction	4,464	2,998	—	2,998	1,466	493	973
Publicly owned facilities	1,204	—	—	—	1,204	246	958
Privately owned facilities	3,260	2,998	—	2,998	262	247	15

Source of funds

bring so many of these scientific advancements within easy reach of every clinical laboratory facility. The quantity, quality, and variety of laboratory testing made available by this combination of talents over the past twenty years can only be described as extraordinary. The hospital laboratory has therefore been cast into a dominant role in the diagnosis and treatment of a large number of disease processes. These advancements are examples of the remarkable capacity of the American free enterprise system to constantly improve its technology and make the benefits widely available. It is a system that must not be dissipated or legislated away.

Because of these developments, laboratory educational opportunities have been expanded. Larger numbers of trained personnel are available to translate this sophisticated technology into direct patient and physician services. In addition to greater emphasis on college and advanced degrees, lower level training programs are producing large numbers of skilled personnel. In most instances, the quality and quantity of education match the technological demands.

Medical education continues to place great importance on modern techniques. As a consequence, physicians have come to rely heavily on laboratory technology in their diagnostic and therapeutic efforts. They recognize that automation and sophisticated technology provide the opportunity for rapid, accurate, and comprehensive patient evaluation. The more recent graduates not only accept these advancements, but also demand their availability.

On the political scene, legislators and bureaucrats are making lively efforts to provide all Americans with "bigger and better" health care. Simultaneously, these same policy makers grope for ways to restrain the seemingly endless spiral of rising health care costs. A review of the massive federal legislation beginning in the 1940s with the Hill-Burton act, and continuing through the current PSRO programs, is more than sufficient to establish the government's impact not only on the construction of health care facilities, but also on the quality of their services.

Of additional impact on this expanded volume of laboratory testing is the recent profusion of malpractice suits against physicians. As a result of these suits large numbers of combative members of the medical profession have initiated such recourse as countersuits; other physicians have abandoned, limited, or relocated their practices. The less disgruntled seek some protection by ordering larger numbers of diagnostic tests. We suspect that the height of the skirmish has passed, but the resulting increased laboratory utilization will not soon be discontinued.

These, then, are the forces we perceive to have accounted most importantly for the growth of the hospital laboratory. It is not expected they will diminish during the foreseeable future. Barring unexpected disclosures of the causes and means of prevention of major diseases, improved care will be sought by greater emphasis on early detection. Laboratory services will no doubt play a major role in these efforts. Research and development shall continue unabated, inevitably followed by the introduction of new products and more sophisticated instruments. More skilled and specialized physicians and laboratory personnel will provide the direct patient benefits so afforded by this advanced technology. Government intrusions on these forthcoming events can only be awaited.

Despite this remarkable growth and such bright prospects, hospital management practices commonly fail to match the levels of skill and efficiency mandated in more competitive business circumstances. The hospital industry has operated essentially within a protected economic environment. Guaranteed cost reimbursement and reckless acquisition of sophisticated equipment without regard for local need have contributed to our inflation woes. With hospital spending accounting for 40 percent of health care expenditures, is it any wonder that two of the most important health bills before Congress are focused on controlling hospital costs?

Much of this lack of managerial expertise can be traced to the early conception of hospitals as charitable institutions where patients were ministered merciful care, all seemed good and nothing was challenged, and financial imbalances were countered by private donations and endowments. The hospital occupied a lofty and austere position. Physicians were respected and their decisions went unquestioned. Alternative facilities essentially were not available. The setting forced little attention on tight management and financial practices. Patient care was a singular concern.

Similarly, the hospital laboratory was solely oriented and occupied by technical responsibilities. Efforts to stay apace of scientific advancements consumed the total energies of the staff and its management responsibilities were neglected. Furthermore, solitary emphasis on analytical skills throughout most laboratory training programs did nothing to correct the problem. Of late, however, and largely out of concern for burgeoning costs, emphasis on the quality of test results is being matched by demands for their more efficient delivery.

In the past several years laboratory journals have become increasingly laden with articles addressing a wide range of management problems. At the same time the professional organizations whose members provide most of the hospital laboratory leadership have recognized these many difficulties and have sponsored attempts to deal with them. Because of their increasing involvement in payment for hospital services, the state and federal governments have actively attempted to legislate performance standards. However, in comparison with other large American businesses, management practices in the hospital and hospital laboratory industries continue to lag severely.

11

What can be done to deal with this extreme example of "success in spite of oneself"? We perceive a need for major efforts to develop greater managerial, operating, and financial skills in the hospital laboratory. It is our judgment that a lack of interest in these matters represents the largest single weakness of most hospital laboratories and must be corrected in order to deal with coming events. This is not a plea for less emphasis on technical skills, only for their more efficient utilization.

The tremendous growth of this sector of the economy has propelled the hospital laboratory to a higher plateau of managerial complexity and responsibility. The subjects to be presented in this text are a response to these developments. They are intended to assist hospital laboratory workers who do not fully perceive the importance of skilled management, operational, and financial practices to the efficient delivery of services. We hope to provide these same persons with greater insight into basic organization concepts. We seek to generate an awareness of total laboratory responsibilities and lend assistance in meeting them. After long neglect, these matters are urgent!

Discussion of test methods, except basic measures for their selection and reliable performance, is omitted. Our concern is not in this area where laboratory personnel are so adequately trained and about which so much has been written. Our concern is rather with management activities, which have been long ignored. It is here that the greatest weaknesses exist, hampering the daily efforts of all or most laboratory workers.

The subjects are purposely presented in their "manual mode," but the reader is encouraged to recognize the frequent potential for computer application. This contemplation of computerization brings us to a major point in planning for future hospital laboratory growth and development. It may represent the single largest opportunity for advancement in the next decade.

Although computers are currently found in many hospital laboratories, it is far from certain that the most meaningful and useful applications have been determined. Any number of these facilities have applied the technology to specimen identification, worksheet generation, cumulative reporting, and on-line data reduction. On too many occasions, however, these practices concern only style, and attending costs cannot be justified by the operational benefits.

We are concerned that more meaningful hospital laboratory computer applications be determined. It is, perhaps, in the subjects to be presented that the greatest use will be found.

We would also like to mention that although the subjects are directed principally at hospital laboratory personnel, the information can be of value to other hospital departments. This requires only that time be taken to deliberate the subjects, personalize the message, and substitute appropriate job titles, equipment, etc. In this event, greater forces might be mobilized in a concerted effort to resolve these many long-ignored and widespread problems.

PART TWO

Modern management concepts

2

PLANNING IN THE HOSPITAL LABORATORY

Planning may be perceived as the methodical selection of a series or set of complementary actions for the purpose of pursuing an improved position. It requires an understanding of the circumstances spawning the plan and a deliberate choice of intermediate positions that best assure the ultimate destination. This fundamental responsibility is critical to the successful operation of the hospital laboratory.

GENERAL PRINCIPLES

Laboratory planning, when diagrammed (Fig. 2-1), is depicted suspended in delicate balance between the sum of the organizational circumstances (operational data) and the ends toward which the efforts are directed (goals). The operational data are required to be constantly current and arranged in manageable units; the mission is pursued by selection of realistic and compatible objectives. The planning is both strategic (identification of goals) and tactical (methods for their accomplishment). Although there are other possible alternative groupings of the operational data, the more detailed discussion of hospital laboratory planning that follows refers to the diagram appearing in Fig. 2-1.

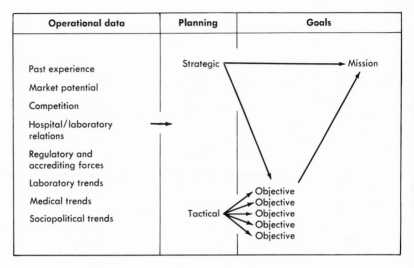

Operational data	Planning	Goals

FIG. 2-1
Essential factors in planning in the hospital laboratory.

LABORATORY GOALS

Mission

A mission is a final and ultimate goal. Its size and scope are determined by the hopes and aspirations of those from whom it takes origin and to whom its achievement provides total and sustaining satisfaction. Missions, if viewed in this context, generally defy accomplishment and permit only pursuit.

Laboratory test results play an important and sometimes singular role in the diagnosis and treatment of many disease processes. When combined with the history, physical examination, X-ray studies, and special procedures, they round out a comprehensive accumulation of data by which sound medical judgments can be made. As with other evaluation modes, they must be provided with professional pride and a keen awareness of their serious impact on the survival and well-being of the patient.

If one accepts the preceding proposals, it is quite apparent that *the mission of every hospital laboratory is the constant provision of timely and accurate test results for the purpose of assisting the physician in the delivery of good patient care.* Pursuit of this mission is greatly assisted by a professional environment where all personnel may learn the highest standards of laboratory medicine and where these standards are recognized and practiced constantly.

Objectives

As shown in Fig. 2-1, laboratory objectives represent the interim goals by which the mission is most logically and effectively pursued. Objectives may be immediate (priorities), intermediate, or long range. Because of the constantly changing status of the operational data and progress of the organization, they require periodic review and updating.

Each laboratory must recognize that identification, documentation, and accomplishment of meaningful and realistic objectives are of major importance to orderly and manageable growth and development. These objectives, like the markers charting long-distance running events, map a well-defined course. Each marker serves as an easily identified and attainable location, arrival at which serves to generate new and determined energies.

OPERATIONAL DATA

Past experience

Past experience, in the context of this presentation, refers to the totality of an organization's awareness based upon the prior observations and participations of its membership. It represents the single most important organizational resource. Because of its importance, thorough and ongoing review and analysis of operational events and personnel persuasions are essential.

As with all input, careful assessments must be made in order to distinguish what is valid from what is not. Some input will represent well-supported conclusions based on accurately recorded data, such as test volume, income and expense figures, and work hours. Much of the input

19

however, is often a loose assortment of impressions and poorly documented appraisals of organizational needs and accomplishments. These latter have no place in the laboratory or any other decision-making process.

The operational data in Fig. 2-1 can be imagined as a constantly undulating and advancing front. If this front derives much of its configuration from the organization's experiences, it is important that these experiences be carefully documented and only the best supported conclusions permitted to influence the decision-making process. This simply assures an exact sighting of each new position and a secure perspective for efficiently and safely negotiating the remaining distance.

Market potential

Market potential may be stated as the known or estimated expenditures for given services in a given locale, or as projections of these expenditures contingent upon specific plans and anticipated developments. These analyses and/or projections are critical to any contemplation of expanded services and, as already stated, include not only a determination of current sales, but also how these sales might be profitably increased with careful strategy.

Although hospital laboratories are not usually run in the same manner as more commercially oriented businesses, they do represent profit centers and promotion and expansion of their services should be considered. This should include orientation of the medical staff to the services available, efforts to more efficiently and effectively deliver these services, the addition of meaningful new procedures, and the solicitation and acquisition of local and regional physician out-patient accounts.

Competition

An analysis of most market potential areas will usually disclose a relatively consistent set of competitive forces. A brief assessment of these forces appears in Table 2-1. It is obvious from this evaluation that efficiencies and availability of out-patient services are of major importance in promoting greater utilization of the hospital's laboratory facilities.

The unwillingness of hospitals and their laboratories to provide the out-patient services so obviously in demand represents the largest single factor contributing to the beginnings and subsequent success of the commercial laboratory industry. To those who inadvertently permitted this occurrence, the information in Table 2-1 should assist in reassessing their position; to those who have purposely avoided providing these services, Table 2-1 calls attention to the not unlikely demands for their availability in the near future.

TABLE 2-1

Assessment of hospital laboratory competition

Competition	Strengths	Weaknesses	Strategy
Physicians' office laboratories	Profitability Patient convenience	Limited range of tests Limited availability Lack of quality control programs	Efficient, comprehensive, and convenient out-patient services Competitive prices
Area hospital laboratories	Must be assessed individually	Must be assessed individually	As above
Commercial laboratories	Good quality Wide range of tests	Inconvenient Impersonal	As above
State health departments	Good quality Small direct cost	Inconvenient Impersonal Slow results	As above PR program (unfair competition)

The current state and federal inquiries into why laboratories in physicians' offices are not required to display the same expertise as hospital laboratories is long overdue. These inquiries are expected to have both short- and long-range impact with no less effect than the insistence on quality control and proficiency testing where they are most needed.

State laboratories continue to be funded by their respective legislatures. In many instances this is for routine tests provided at minimal or no charge. Greater efforts are needed to divert the full resources of these facilities to assisting and complementing the services of the hospital laboratory rather than providing unfair competition at the expense of the unknowing taxpayer.

Hospital/laboratory relations

The management and operation of the hospital laboratory have all too frequently resulted in a host of difficulties between those responsible for providing its services and those accountable for administering overall hospital policy. Many of the problems can be attributed to a less than full and mutual appreciation of the difficulties and problems that attend these major areas of responsibility, and the frequently poor or selfish planning with which the relationship is established and conducted.

Contributing to these difficulties is the aberrant and bizarre configuration of most hospital organizations, which resulted from the unorthodox relationship of the medical staff to the remainder of the structure. Although this group has less-than-full organizational involvement, it exercises a major influence on delivery of services. In no other organization does an "outside" force have such impact on internal operations. We liken this situation to a large and difficult-to-repair hernia (Fig. 2-2).

Because of the potential that these and other hospital organizational peculiarities have for serious disruption of

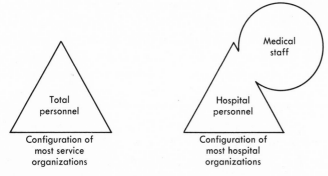

FIG. 2-2

Diagrammatic demonstration of the unorthodox configuration of most hospital organizations. The area occupied by the medical staff represents not necessarily numbers, but rather authority.

smooth and effective operational relations, it is essential that authority and responsibilities are carefully delineated. Firm definition of these relationships is particularly representative of the importance of well documented operational data by which realistic sightings of laboratory objectives can be made and secure and confident plans formulated.

Regulatory and accrediting forces

Expenditures for laboratory services constitute a large segment of the current multibillion dollar American health care "program." Primarily because of this expense, but also because of gross violations of public trust and the relative ease of scrutiny, the entire laboratory industry has been subjected to a large and ever-increasing number of regulations and performance standards. This phenomenon characterizes the constraints currently being imposed on all providers of medical services.

Although we do not argue against well-conceived and realistic standards by which the quality of performance is

23

objectively measured, we are very concerned about the arbitrariness of many of these standards, their mysterious origins and bureaucratic support, and the frequency with which the objectives they seemingly are attempting to achieve—namely quality and cost control—are in such direct, entangled, and frustrating conflict.

To better illustrate the extent to which regulatory constraints are influencing every hospital laboratory, an abbreviated list of these forces is presented here. With minimal effort this almost comical docket of legislation and private and bureaucratic agencies could easily be expanded.

```
CLIA, 1967
CLIA, 1978 (pending)
CDC
BQA
BHI
OSHA
FDA
CAP (I&A)
CAP (PTS)
ASCP
AABB
JCAH
NAACLS
PTS
```

There is little doubt that the relative strengths of these forces shall change in the coming years. Despite the efforts of the still existing private laboratory sector, greater governmental intrusions are anticipated. Whatever the outcome, all forces must be recognized and anticipated during any serious efforts to plan the well-being of the hospital laboratory.

A trend may be defined as a series of events constituting a pattern that suggests both its origin and probabilities for continuation. Laboratory trends serve as valuable indicators of consensus thinking within the industry and, as such, provide an important means by which one's own thinking and practices may be influenced.

Laboratory trends may support or reverse personal persuasions and anticipations. They may raise doubt concerning those people contributing to their occurrence. Trends are not always based on valid observations and conclusions; nor are they always of long duration. As a matter of fact, they often are only stylish and, like styles in other areas, frequently have a short or seasonal appeal. Foolish and unnecessary efforts can often be avoided if management refrains from initiating practices justified solely on conformity. A particularly good example of this point will be found in the discussion of analytical quality control (Chapter 8).

However, management personnel should be constantly aware of the swings and moods in national and regional laboratory thinking. In conjunction with one's own circumstances and experience, knowledge of trends can contribute significantly to providing more secure and effective delineation of organizational direction.

Laboratory trends

The pattern of test requests is a useful indicator of the relative value with which the physician perceives the wide range of laboratory services. Any assessment of changes in laboratory request patterns, particularly as they relate to stated needs for new procedures, should include an assessment of improved disease evaluation and the probabilities of sustained utilization. Examples of both long- and short-term usage of new tests can be cited including the frustrations and unnecessary expense that accompany the latter.

Additional impact on hospital laboratory services are

Medical trends

25

trends in the location of new practices and the relocation of old. The best example of this might be the tendency to cluster physicians' offices in the immediate vicinity of the hospital, which results in greater utilization of its outpatient facilities. Another occurrence is the employment of full-time emergency room physicians and its effect on laboratory staffing requirements.

Perhaps the greatest impact has been the emphasis on early disease detection and the variety of laboratory services employed in such an effort. In the absence of any realistic expectations of solutions to the cause or prevention of these diseases, this trend is expected to continue.

Sociopolitical trends

Major changes in the operation of hospital laboratories are arising out of the sociopolitical trends that have long existed and are now gathering increased momentum. The loud espousing of the benefits of national health insurance by politicians and legislators echoes the desire by the public for total change in our health care delivery system.

Events that have already affected hospital laboratories include the legislation of equal job opportunities and legalization of unions in nonprofit institutions. Less intimately related to the legislative efforts has been the behavior of our nation's "free spirits" resulting in an entirely new drug toxicology industry. Yet to be formalized are the "solutions" to the maldistribution of medical services and final plans for the centralization of clinical laboratory services.

Contemplation of these and other previously mentioned forces on the delivery of hospital laboratory services is both engaging and repelling. This dilemma arises out of a willingness to accept greater overall organizational efforts as a means of improving health care and a fear that the expense and accompanying arbitrary bureaucratic standards will surely and irreparably curtail efficiencies, originality, and desire.

PLANNING

Strategic planning

We intentionally followed a circuitous route in arriving at the ultimate task of examining the planning process. The purpose was to first call attention to the variety of data that must be considered and to lend clearer definition of goals and the sequence for their attainment. We may now give thought to the translation of aspirations into reality.

Strategic planning is conceptual and deals with the sweeping question of *what to do*. As indicated in Fig. 2-1, it is concerned with identification of the mission and of those objectives that will permit its most efficient pursuit. Effective strategic planning requires an insight into total operational capabilities and a keen awareness of all opposing forces. It is a function of upper level supervisory personnel with final authority and responsibility vested in the laboratory director.

This portion of the planning process must be conducted in accordance with each laboratory's own set of circumstances and operating style, precluding any meaningful discussion of specific methodology. Let it only be said that it requires a keen recognition of all internal and external factors bearing on the laboratory's position and is enhanced by an environment conducive to an open exchange of ideas.

Tactical planning

Tactical planning implies action and deals with the method(s) for achieving the goals identified in the strategic planning process. It often requires an operational or technical skill and is generally a logical responsibility of the supervisory staff.

These responsibilities can be wasteful of organizational time and resources unless care is exercised in selecting those persons whose talents most closely match with the task. A keen awareness of the interests and abilities of the laboratory staff is important in making these assignments.

27

CONCLUSIONS   Planning is an integral part and immediate forerunner of all daily activity, and is generally conducted with aplomb and success. However, because of the routineness of these activities, the inherent requirements of this planning process too often go unrecognized. As a consequence, less-than-satisfactory results are often achieved when the planning becomes more involved and complex.

This chapter has been an attempt to identify and isolate the fundamental components of this major responsibility. It is intended to assist the reader in understanding their importance and relationships and in utilizing this greater insight in his or her own planning efforts. To further emphasize the importance of the subject, we quote Goethe:

> To plan and not act is futile;
> to act and not plan is fatal!

3

ORGANIZING AND STAFFING THE HOSPITAL LABORATORY

Organization denotes an effort to divide total operations into the size and types of units by which efficient and effective services are best assured and needs and weaknesses most easily identified. It is a major management responsibility for the purpose of securing a united and cohesive performance.

In most hospitals all laboratory services traditionally have been assigned to one department. These assignments stem largely from pathology residency programs that train physicians in all or most of the medical laboratory fields; these physicians are therefore available full- or part-time to direct the delivery of these services. Contributing to this arrangement is the dearth of clinicians with either time or interest to justify transfer of these services closer to the patient setting.

Because of the teaching and investigative roles of the full-time staff members of a university hospital, other divisions of responsibility may be found in these institutions. Special (and sometimes not so special) laboratory services are often considered to be most effectively provided by the clinical departments that utilize these services exclusively or most frequently.

For this discussion, however, we are assuming that one

hospital department has total responsibility for providing laboratory services. Given this usual method of departmentalization, we will reflect for a moment on the further division of these services. The point we wish to examine is not the types of services, but the classification of the operating units generating these services.

It must be understood that despite their proximity, hospital laboratory services (chemistry, hematology, microbiology, etc.) have little else in common. They are distinct laboratory fields requiring considerably different education and training of personnel. Each is a unique discipline embodying large volumes of technical data and employing considerably different analytical techniques and instrumentation.

For these reasons, it is only reasonable that each of the operating divisions be recognized for the scientifically independent and autonomous units they are—laboratories! This would immediately identify the organization to which they belong as a "Department of Laboratories." The acceptance of this reasoning would alleviate our long frustration with such misnomers as "laboratory," "lab," "pathology," etc., and would distinguish these facilities for finally having learned their proper names.

With regard to hospital laboratory staffing, the sheer growth and diversity of laboratory services clearly demonstrate the need for specialization of personnel. The field of laboratory medicine has expanded too broadly and developed too large a body of data for any realistic expectation that a sufficient degree of expertise can be obtained in more than one of its disciplines. Despite these obvious factors, brisk and disconcerting efforts persist to train and employ "all purpose" laboratory workers. The entire matter requires close attention by those developing and conducting the various training programs and is an important consideration during attempts to staff the hospital laboratory.

Efficient and effective selection, grouping, and utilization of personnel constitute a major responsibility, written policies for which are essential for several reasons. First, and most importantly, a written policy requires of the leadership a careful and detailed analysis of all personnel needs and interrelationships and one would hope a subsequent awareness of exactly what these are. Second, it provides all personnel with written verification of the deliberations and decisions and the specific roles they are expected to fill. In this context, documented policies refer to a table of organization, job descriptions, and job specifications, all of which are essential to a solidly and securely structured organization.

TABLE OF ORGANIZATION

A table of organization is a diagram (chart) that identifies the major operational units of an organization and their attending job positions. The positions of greater responsibility are located at the top while those of lesser accountability appear on correspondingly lower levels. Lines have been inserted to clearly indicate the channels of communication. These lines are straight! They run vertically and horizontally and begin and terminate in precise positions. They complete a graphic demonstration of the total organization including the rank and relationship of all its parts.

From an operational standpoint, the table of organization is the single most concise representation of the organization and provides an important means of managing and monitoring all of its activities. It also provides the membership an understanding of their station and how they relate to one another. (For a hypothetical hospital laboratory table of organization, see Table 3-1.)

JOB DESCRIPTIONS

Job descriptions are written declarations of given job positions. They may be done in a variety of formats, but in all

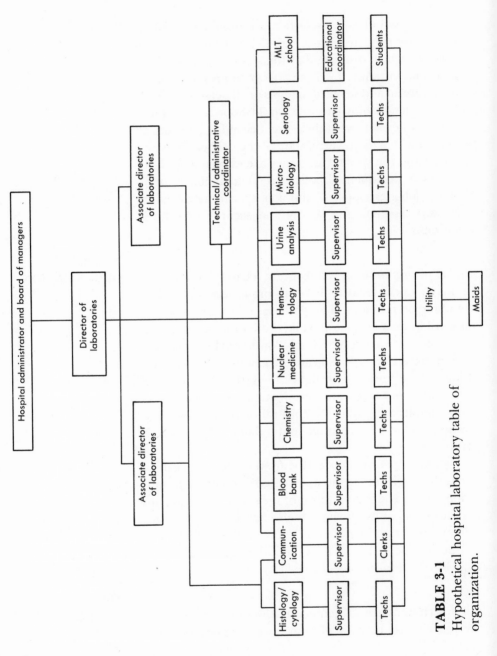

TABLE 3-1
Hypothetical hospital laboratory table of organization.

instances they must clearly affirm each duty and responsibility. Job descriptions supplement the table of organization by providing definition to all positions. They force the leadership to identify operational duties and responsibilities, and they provide a means of avoiding unnecessary duplication and overlapping of efforts.

Well-conceived job descriptions assure that all operational duties and responsibilities have been assigned and that employees know precisely what is expected of them. They assist with equitable salary classifications and lend orderliness to job performance.

Some people contend, however, that job descriptions are unrealistic and ineffective. It is argued that they are restrictive and burdensome and rarely achieve desired results. Finally, one hears, job descriptions usually receive only token recognition and, when it is decided that they meet with commonsense preconceptions of the job, they are usually filed away and forgotten.

In response to these criticisms, we emphasize that job planning is a major managerial responsibility. It requires assessments and decisions the merits of which can be decided only after the job descriptions are written and analyzed. Without this thoughtful and methodical sequence, vague and conflicting perceptions emerge, and management by crises and erratic notions becomes a distinct possibility.

Organizations attempting to operate in this manner are generally observed to be disorganizations. Furthermore, when formulating plans for the efficient performance of job duties, management personnel must avoid feigning sound organizational principles. Rather, they must carefully assess a variety of options and select those that most effectively utilize people's time and efforts and challenge each person to improve the quality of his or her performance. (For hypothetical job descriptions, see Appendix A.)

JOB
SPECIFICATIONS

Job specifications represent the requirements for employment in a given job. The format consists of a set of factors or parameters that bear significantly on all or most positions and a corresponding set of prerequisites developed specifically for the job(s) under consideration. These specifications provide the organization with the personnel requirements considered to match most efficiently with the demands of each job. They are invaluable in recruitment because they eliminate the uncertainties as to just who and what are sought.

The factors alluded to include education, experience, and a number of other considerations relating to the mental and physical aspects of the job and its environment. For most hospital laboratory positions, the education factor demands the greatest deliberation because of its impact on the organization's attainable level of sophistication. It is unfortunate that the salary constraints of most hospitals limit the levels to which so many aspire. It is a problem that laboratory directors must address more thoughtfully and forcefully in the future.

Job specifications help management to articulate the personnel standards of the organization; they are critical to successful laboratory staffing. In addition to their impact on professional attainment, the specifications assist in reducing the wasteful and self-defeating problems of personnel over- and underutilization by providing a closer and more cost-effective match between the difficulties of the job and the workers to whom the job is assigned. (For hypothetical hospital laboratory job specifications, see Appendix A.)

WORK
SCHEDULES

The uninterrupted demands for daily hospital laboratory services dictate a thorough and ongoing analysis of personnel needs throughout each twenty-four hour period. The unpredictability of disease processes and the frequent attending need for urgent test results add significantly to the importance of carefully planned work schedules.

The arbitrary but firmly established practice of eight-hour shifts serves as the usual method of dividing each twenty-four–hour period. The staffing of these shifts depends upon demand and the availability of personnel to meet this demand. Because of request patterns, the largest number of personnel are scheduled during the first eight-hour period while second and third shifts are staffed with far fewer people, generally for the purpose of providing services only in case of unexpected and critical illness.

Because of the uncertainty and inconsistency with which emergencies occur, chronic and nagging problems can arise because of the costliness of overstaffing and the delays and ineffectiveness caused by understaffing. The frequency with which second and third shift personnel are observed to be either too busy or not busy enough, is sufficient reason to deliberate this problem.

Realistic increases in second and third shift staffing for the purpose of providing both emergency and some routine services should be considered. Such increases may diminish or eliminate the problems of insufficient personnel during times of heavy emergency workloads while providing on all other occasions many nonurgent services that are customarily delayed until the following day.

State and federal regulatory agencies will undoubtedly press for more efficient utilization of personnel as a means of shortening hospital stays and reducing cost. More effective scheduling of laboratory personnel as a means of assisting with these economy measures thus becomes a meaningful objective.

PERSONNEL REQUIREMENTS AND WORKLOAD MEASUREMENTS

Because personnel constitute the largest laboratory cost, strong efforts must be made to assure their most effective utilization. Fundamental considerations of personnel numbers, distribution, and responsibilities and the value of carefully selected personnel qualifications are discussed previously under Table of Organization, Job Descriptions, and Job Specifications.

Given the best matching of employees with jobs, assessments of efficiency of performance are of benefit. Because of the great variety of laboratory testing, standardized measurements of effort are required. These provide a method for recording and comparing the workload in all areas and, when related appropriately to manhours, become a means for assessing productivity.

Such a method may be found in *A Workload Recording Method for Clinical Laboratories,** third edition, 1976. The method is modeled after the system developed in Canada and published as the *Canadian Schedule of Unit Values for Clinical Laboratory Procedures,*† 1970.

Work units are assigned each procedure by determining the average total time (technical, clerical, etc.) required for performance. Each unit is equivalent to one minute of time exclusive of specimen collection and measurements of controls, duplicates, and repeats. Recording the workload requires an initial tally of the number of procedures performed and their subsequent multiplication by the work units so assigned. These assignments must be individualized for each laboratory, but because of the standardization of so much methodology, many of the values may be taken directly from the publications mentioned before.

After the workload is completed in work units, an additional computation of the relationship of this workload to the manhours required for its performance provides a useful estimate of productivity.

$$\frac{\text{Total work units}}{\text{Total work hours}} = \text{Work units/hour}$$

*College of American Pathologists, 230 North Michigan Avenue, Chicago, Illinois 60601.
†Statistics, Canada Health and Welfare Division, Institutions Section, Ottawa, Canada.

Obviously, the closer the work units per hour approach 60, the greater the productivity. Comparisons by area, shifts, etc., can be made and limits of acceptable performance easily established. When these are not appropriate, corrective action is taken.

A number of factors may explain variations in productivity from one laboratory area to another. A major reason is variations in the ability to batch the workload. As an example, the reader is encouraged to contemplate the work patterns of histology and cytology laboratories where productivity measurements are among the highest. In any event, efforts to avoid random and single test performance, without compromising patient services, contribute significantly to efficient utilization of personnel and resources.

4

DIRECTING AND SUPERVISING THE HOSPITAL LABORATORY

GENERAL PRINCIPLES

Directing may be considered a display of methods and means for getting from one location to another. In management parlance, the relocation points are often identified as objectives and the instructions for arrival as policies and procedures. For greatest effectiveness, directions must be written, comprehensive, current, clearly stated and reinforced by discussion and example.

Supervision is a critical adjunct to directing and entails responsibility for assuring that policies and procedures are followed. It includes an understanding and agreement with established goals and an active role in their formulation and achievement.

Such demanding responsibilities require an enthusiasm for and a convincing presentation of the organizational aims. The director or supervisor must be able to persuade personnel that the success of these endeavors is equivalent to the success of each of the participants. Careful observers will usually conclude that an organization's achievements are closely allied with the quality of this leadership.

LEADERSHIP QUALITIES

Although leadership is acknowledged to be a fundamental organizational principle, analysis of its requirements is fraught with difficulties. The closest scrutiny is unlikely to divulge any consistent set of qualities that characterize all persons occupying the same or similar positions. Widely varying interests, skills, background, and convictions are readily observed among successful laboratory directors and supervisors. Shortcomings in one area are overcome by great strengths in another.

How are these differences in leadership qualities accounted for? Are they innate or acquired? Can one be considered superior to another? If so, what is the evidence? For example, can it be established that a given strength generates greater organizational effectiveness? We can, of course, recite the familiar phrases: "the willingness to accept responsibility" or "the drive to get things done," but these are simplistic and do little to explain the total leadership phenomenon.

If, indeed, the existence of a common set or even dominant leadership characteristics is uncertain, might there simply be fortuitous events that unite the leader and followers and inspire the efforts of both? This is doubtful. Even if a foreign menace resulting in a national unity is cited, it is unlikely that a counterpart will be found in the organizational matters with which we are concerned.

In attempting to analyze the leadership phenomenon, we must recognize at least four basic factors: (1) the abilities of the leader; (2) the characteristics of the followers; (3) the nature and mission of the organization; and (4) the social, economic, and political setting within which the organization operates.

The first factor, leadership abilities, is worthy of additional comment. It is presented best as leadership styles, which, although easily recognized, are not always so readily understood.

LEADERSHIP STYLES

A hospital laboratory is essentially a system of human relationships in which the members are united by goals and expectations. Directors and supervisors occupy positions within this network and their patterns of influence materially affect outcome. Differences in these patterns (leadership styles) are as varied as in other professions, but experience will generally identify several that prevail.

The first evolves from a *conviction of the merits of decentralized authority*. It places major importance on the delegation of responsibility. Leaders who use this style are concerned with achievement, but seek it through planned participation. They are highly concerned with the organizational structure through which the work proceeds. The leader points the organization's direction, initiates movement, and provides the motivation by which momentum is self-energized and accelerated by each of its parts. Communication is conducted through a well-defined chain of command that encourages an exchange and integration of ideas, but channels this input in an orderly and uniform manner.

In this style the concept of authority is vertical with positions of increasing and decreasing accountability. A manager who uses this style attempts to influence others by suggesting ideas and provoking thoughtful reaction. He or she sets logical and realistic goals and seeks their accomplishment through full but structured participation. The view of those using this style is long ranged, perhaps idealistic, and supported by a capacity to strive for meaningful accomplishments.

The strengths of the style relate largely to the consistencies of the operations and roles of the participants. The relationship of the individual to the organization permits each person to maintain and build upon a strong sense of self-esteem and the opportunity to actively participate and contribute to a process of orderly and methodical accomplishment.

The style also has weaknesses. The major flaws are: (1) if one part performs poorly, the entire system is jeopardized, i.e., there is no self-correcting mechanism; and (2) there is possibly a sense of isolation by the lower ranks. These flaws can be avoided if the leaders recognize the importance of all organizational input and their responsibility for assuring it is never obstructed or distorted.

The second common leadership style is based on the *concept of centralized authority* and the importance of the leader knowing all operational details. It places little value on an orderly chain of command and condones a variety of information sources in the name of an "open door" policy.

Managers who use this style view all authority to be concentrated at the very top. This centralization of power controls activity and communication at the highest level and, with descent into the lower organizational ranks, individuals are increasingly passive. This is viewed by some as harmful on the grounds that natural human development is from passivity to activity.

In this style singular authority is held to be of greater importance to group achievement than the design or structure of its organization. Most workers are perceived as having little capacity to either develop or contribute. Only one-way communication is generated and there are sufficiently tight controls so that the resulting personnel behavior is made to confirm the initial perception.

The strengths of such a style include an assurance that authority is vested in only one person and actions may be taken quickly and decisively. It avoids lengthy discussions and deliberations in which subordinates might come to conclusions far removed from those already reached and probably acted upon by the leader. This style is further supported by the observation that organizational vitality and achievement are rarely generated by more than a few individuals with the unique capacity for innovation and the initiative and determination to make things move.

The weakness of such a style is the risk of having insecure, uncertain, and restless personnel who have little assurance of a consistent role or set of responsibilities. An unwillingness or inability to contribute to their full potential is the end result. The capabilities of the organization become solely the capabilities of the leader. Growth and development are thwarted by less than full and active participation. Furthermore, with increasing organizational size, singular authority becomes increasingly difficult; there may be crippling voids and lack of attention which will ultimately require major and disruptive managerial revisions.

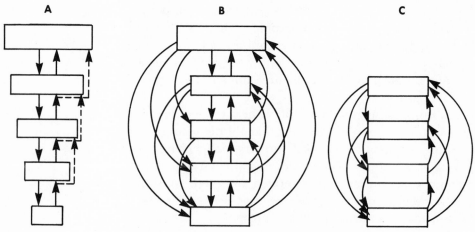
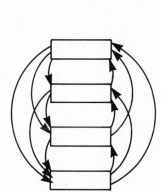

FIG. 4-1

Diagrammatic presentation of three leadership styles commonly used in the hospital laboratory. *Diagram A* demonstrates delegation of authority and responsibility through a chain of command that follows an orderly and consistent pathway. Persons at all levels of the organization are kept constantly informed and involved. Alternative routes are available only after the main pathway is traveled and determined to harbor an impasse. *Diagram B* shows the generation of motion in an assortment of directions. Because staff members are uncertain of their authority and responsibility, their participation in the organization is likely to be ineffective. *Diagram C* is self-explanatory.

A discussion of hospital leadership styles should not be concluded without brief mention of one not infrequently observed. It is best identified as leadership by absenteeism or inattention and is cited only for the purpose of condemning its practice. (See Fig. 4-1 for a diagrammatic expression of the three leadership styles.)

LEADERSHIP RESPONSIBILI- TIES

- To formulate and document policies and procedures that are constantly current and relevant to effective pursuit of laboratory goals.
- To effectively communicate these plans to all personnel.
- To provide efficient means for assuring compliance with policies and procedures.
- To encourage a free flow and exchange of ideas through all levels of the organization.
- To assure an awareness by all personnel of current trends and practices in the delivery of hospital laboratory services.
- To develop and maintain effective relations with the medical staff and hospital administration for assuring an open exchange of the needs and concerns of all parties.

LEADERSHIP METHODS

- To develop and constantly update all laboratory procedures and policies by preparation of appropriate manuals.
- To schedule and conduct periodic meetings with staff for discussion and review of policies and procedures.
- To delegate responsibility for efficiently monitoring compliance with policies and procedures.
- To conduct periodic meetings with laboratory staff to encourage innovative thinking and improvements in service.

- To fully support and generously budget for a meaningful laboratory continuing education program.
- To assure awareness of the laboratory mission by requiring that appropriate personnel attend all hospital and medical staff meetings that call for laboratory representation.

THE LEADERSHIP DILEMMA

A leadership position is often a vulnerable one. A leader faces risks and uncertainties resulting from his or her responsibilities and the scrutiny and influences of others. The role is very often singular and solitary. It is both demanding and compelling and frequently rewarded only by knowing that one's efforts make a difference in the course of events.

The wisdom of their plans and decisions is of constant concern to leaders. Contributing to the concern are the time intervals between initiation of action and observation of results and also the reliability of the feedback. A leader's fears of uncertainty and failure are often accompanied by feelings of inadequate authority and the need to avoid personal inertia. The degree of interdependence and the polarity of leading and being led must be inwardly resolved. How much being liked is compatible with effective authority is a recurrent problem.

Positions of leadership hold authority, with responsibilities that demand judgments bearing significantly on the lives of others. The discontent of subordinates and the implementing of strategy to help them mature and develop can be stressful. Recognizing and satisfying their need for identity and resolving differences among diverse interest groups are not without difficulty. Assisting persons to avoid technical obsolescence demands time and effort. Rivalries must be resolved and balances between cooperation and competition established.

These are just a few of the problems of leadership; they

are often distinguished by the controversy and the variety
of opinions with which they are surrounded. The difficulties of leaders, perhaps, may be best summarized by the
idea that authority is derived from a freedom of action and
exemption from accountability. It can suffer, however, by a
forfeiture of dignity and individuality by the followers. On
the other hand, a lack of authority, with freedom and
equality generously distributed among the membership,
runs the extreme risk of organizational immobility and
ineffectiveness. The leadership dilemma can only be resolved by identifying the appropriate balance between
these two extremes.

PART THREE

Modern operating concepts

5

COMMUNICATION

Communication is the indication of a happening, thought, idea, concept, question, or need. It is most frequently conducted by written or spoken word, but may be conveyed by gestures, lack of gestures, manner of dress, personal appearance, and general behavior.

Because of the growing interdependency of people in modern society, communication is essential for survival. Despite its obvious importance and the many convenient and sophisticated methods of delivery, errors and weaknesses are common with undesirable consequences that range from minor to catastrophic. For these reasons in general and the patient's well being in particular, every laboratory worker must understand the principles and methods by which communication is correctly conducted.

Sophisticated modern hospital care demands that a variety of specialty services and expertise be constantly available. The frequency with which such services must be quickly mobilized requires organized and coordinated efforts between and among their providers. The effectiveness of these efforts is obviously dependent upon well-conceived and conscientiously conducted interdepartmental communication.

The following recommendations are suggested as standards to be constantly met or exceeded:
- Be courteous at all times.
- Speak distinctly and in a pleasant tone of voice.
- Be certain all questions and answers are clearly understood.
- Do not answer questions about which there is uncertainty; consult resources of department (immediate supervisor, manuals, etc.).
- Do not allow delay in answering telephone.
- Never leave telephone unattended after call is received; if placed on "hold," reassure caller at frequent intervals that attempt is being made to complete connection.
- When receiving calls, initiate conversation with "Good morning (Good afternoon, Good evening), Department of Laboratories."
- When transferring calls, inform person of caller's name and department.
- When making calls, preface remarks with name and department.
- Be certain all written or typed reports are neat, legible, and accurate; also that they are dated and initialed or signed.

INTRADEPARTMENTAL COMMUNICATION

Communication is probably always better within a department than between or among departments. Reasons for this include proximity, similar education, related duties, and common goals among coworkers. Because of the closer relationships, constant opportunity is afforded for enhancing the quality of laboratory services. The following recommendations are suggested as standards to be met or exceeded:
- Know the department's table of organization and all communication channels so indicated.
- Be certain of job description and all duties set forth.

- Minimize conversation unrelated to job duties.
- Confer messages by memo if face-to-face or telephone communication is not possible.
- Maintain effective contact with members of all shifts.
- Be constantly alert to the posting of all schedules and notices.

PUBLIC RELATIONS

Although laboratory personnel are not as well recognized as many other providers of health care, good relations with the public and other health care professionals are in the laboratory's best interests. These dealings can be successful if laboratory employees are aware of the importance of harmonious dealings with others. These responsibilities are only met by sincere concern for the needs of others and a genuine attempt to be of assistance.

Included among the daily contacts of hospital laboratory workers are patients, physicians, nurses, salesmen, and other hospital and nonhospital personnel. On all occasions a considerate and confident bearing must be maintained. Considerable time and energy are required to establish a laboratory organization that commands the respect and confidence of the people who use the services. There is no reason why any laboratory employee should not understand this effort or should fail on any occasion to contribute to its success.

Patients

Laboratory workers must constantly recognize that most patients with whom contacts are made have some degree of illness and discomfort about which their physician has expressed concern. Furthermore, these people are in strange surroundings and may suffer embarrassments and even indignities. They are assigned identification numbers and are subjected to unfamiliar and disquieting questions, examinations, treatments, and assorted other disturbing

51

variations from their normal routine. They are apprehensive, insecure, frightened, and, not infrequently, threatened with extinction. Caution must be taken to remember that these patients are *people* not numbers or tests—people in need of assistance. Laboratory personnel must be considerate and understanding of the patient's disadvantage.

Physicians

The ultimate responsibility for the patient's well-being rests directly and singularly with the physician. This is a serious and demanding role that cannot be understood by any person who has not occupied the same position. The large assortment of clinical problems and the unpredictability with which they occur frequently create a need for a range of laboratory services at various times and with various degrees of urgency. Only the physician can decide when tests are needed. Requests for services must not be met by complaints from laboratory personnel concerning inconvenient timing and/or volume.

The sole laboratory response must be prompt acknowledgement of the desired services and their efficient and effective provision. Polite questions and suggestions are not out of order, but the frequency with which undesirable attitudes by laboratory workers are observed is disturbing. Unless they can accept and enjoy a support role and develop an enthusiasm for satisfying physician and patient needs under all circumstances, these laboratory personnel should find employment outside the hospital laboratory.

Nursing personnel

Nursing staff duties represent the hub of hospital patient care from which the needs for additional services are constantly generated. Because of the frequency with which these needs necessitate a laboratory response, a cooperative and coordinated relationship between the nursing and laboratory departments is imperative. The success of such

Text continued on p. 69.

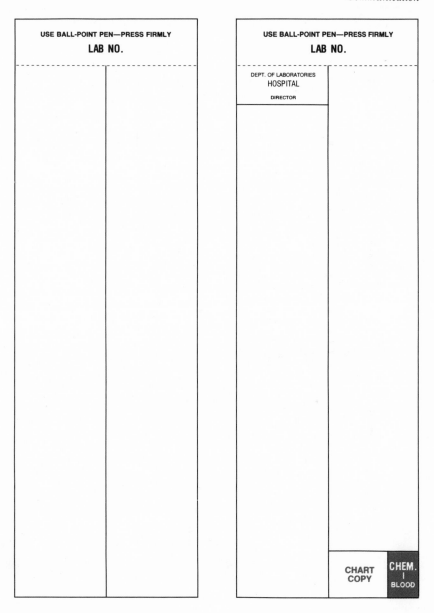

FIG. 5-1
Vertical positioning of 3 by 9¼ inch request/report form divided lengthwise in half.

FIG. 5-2
Request/report form with color coding of chart copy and identification of the facility and its laboratory director.

53

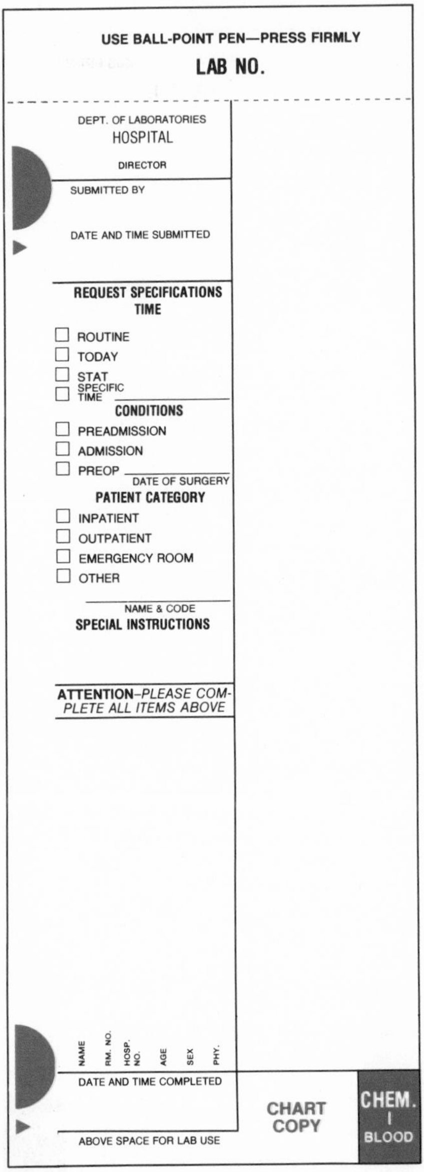

FIG. 5-3
Request/report form with insertion of request information in left column.

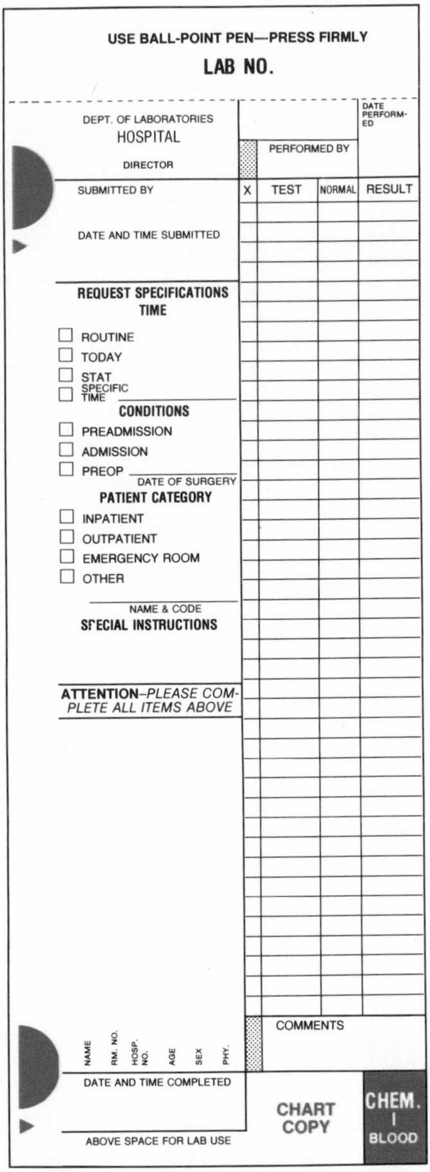

FIG. 5-4
Request/report form with provisions for insertion of report information in right column.

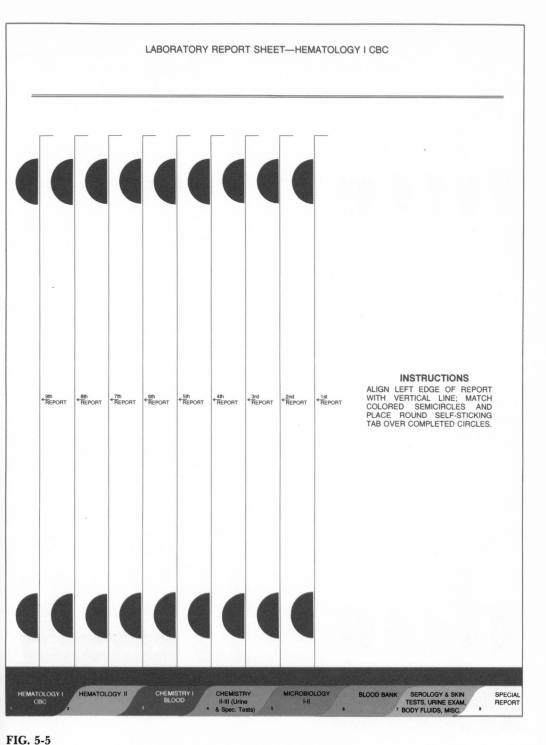

FIG. 5-5

8½ by 11 inch attachment sheets with colored tabs, names of reports to be attached, numbers that read consecutively from left to right, and instructions for affixing reports.

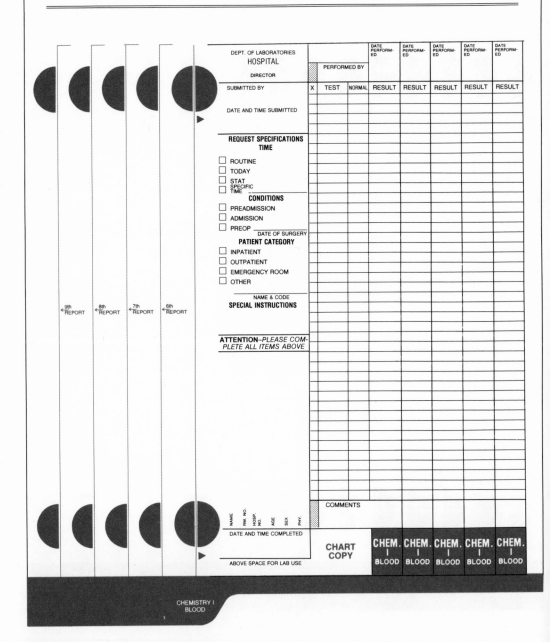

FIG. 5-6
Attachment of reports by name and color with prominent display of the dates of test performance.

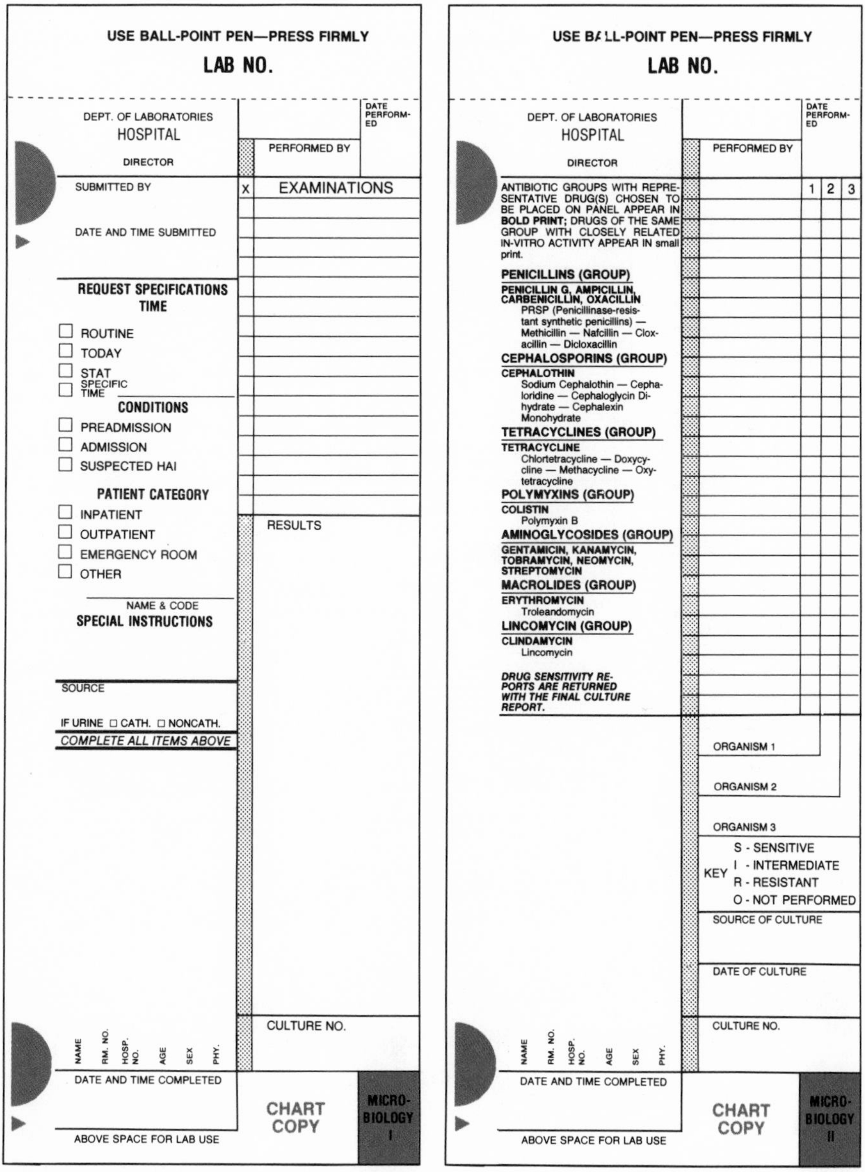

FIG. 5-7
Variations in microbiology reports from standard format.

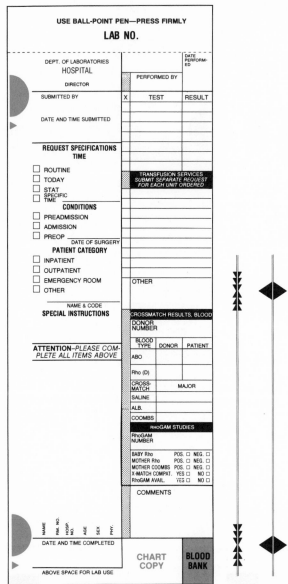

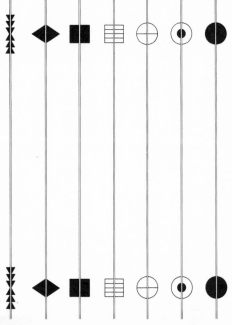

FIG. 5-8
Slight variations from standard format in right column of blood bank report.

FIG. 5-9
Variety of matching configurations for precise alignment of reports.

58

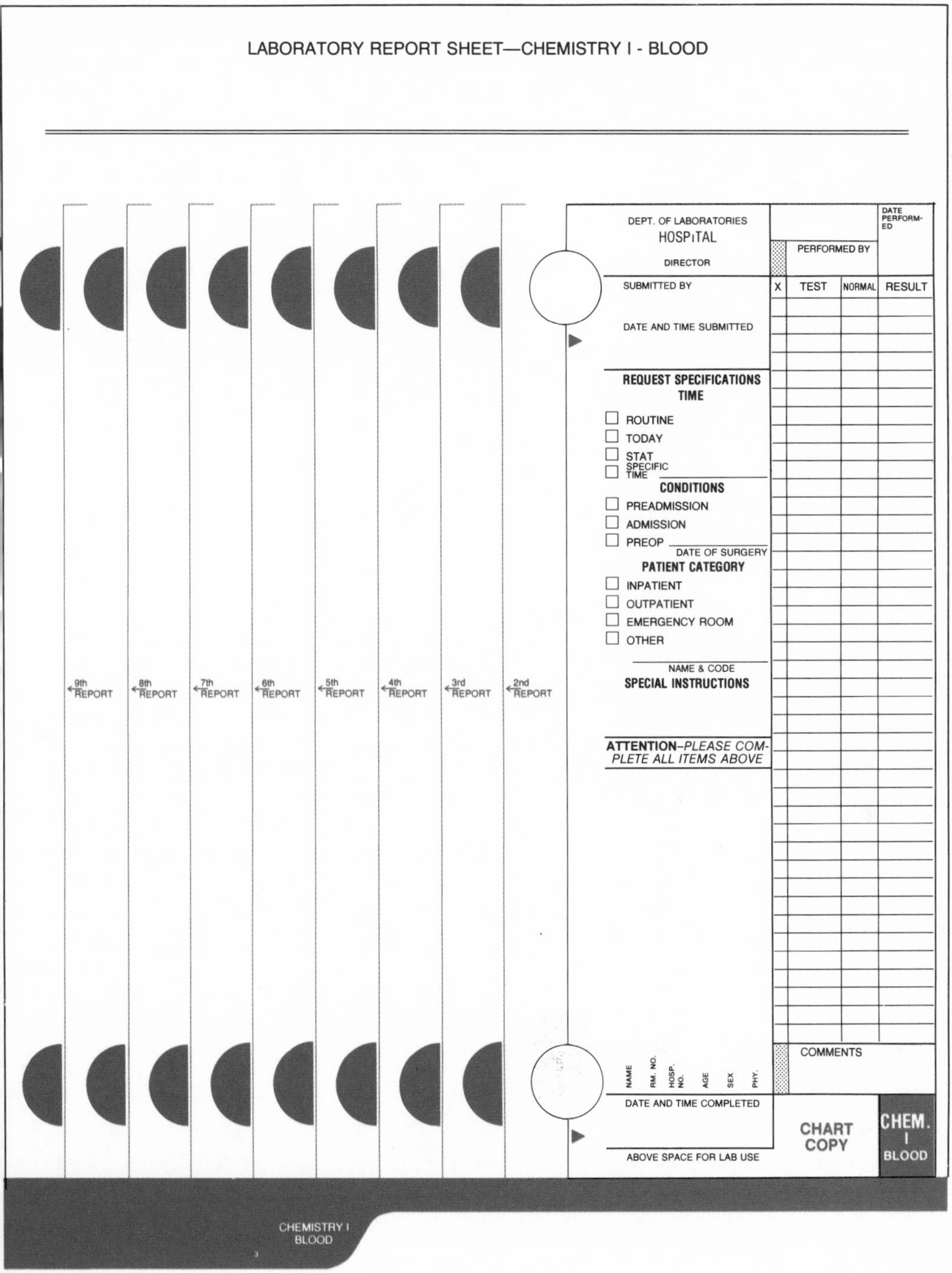

LABORATORY REPORT SHEET—CHEMISTRY I - BLOOD

DEPT. OF LABORATORIES
HOSPITAL
DIRECTOR

| | | DATE PERFORM-ED |
| | PERFORMED BY | |

SUBMITTED BY

DATE AND TIME SUBMITTED

X	TEST	NORMAL	RESULT

REQUEST SPECIFICATIONS
TIME

☐ ROUTINE
☐ TODAY
☐ STAT
☐ SPECIFIC TIME

CONDITIONS

☐ PREADMISSION
☐ ADMISSION
☐ PREOP _____ DATE OF SURGERY

PATIENT CATEGORY

☐ INPATIENT
☐ OUTPATIENT
☐ EMERGENCY ROOM
☐ OTHER

NAME & CODE
SPECIAL INSTRUCTIONS

ATTENTION—*PLEASE COM-PLETE ALL ITEMS ABOVE*

9th REPORT 8th REPORT 7th REPORT 6th REPORT 5th REPORT 4th REPORT 3rd REPORT 2nd REPORT

NAME RM. NO. HOSP. NO. AGE SEX PHY.

COMMENTS

DATE AND TIME COMPLETED

ABOVE SPACE FOR LAB USE

CHART COPY

CHEM. I BLOOD

CHEMISTRY I BLOOD

FIG. 5-10
Attachment of report by inexpensive "permanent" self-adhesive tabs with provisions for an eight additional attachments.

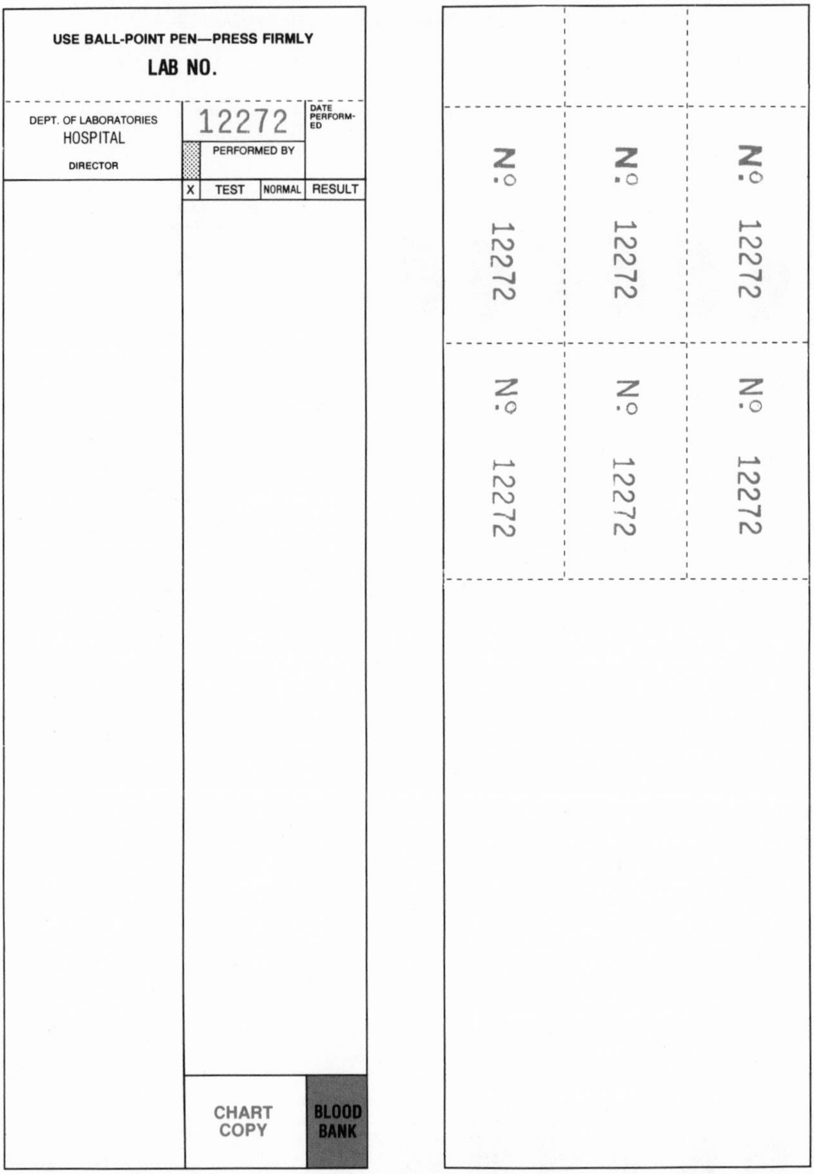

FIG. 5-11

Prenumbered request/report form with identically numbered gummed labels attached to the back of the forms for convenient and inexpensive specimen identification.

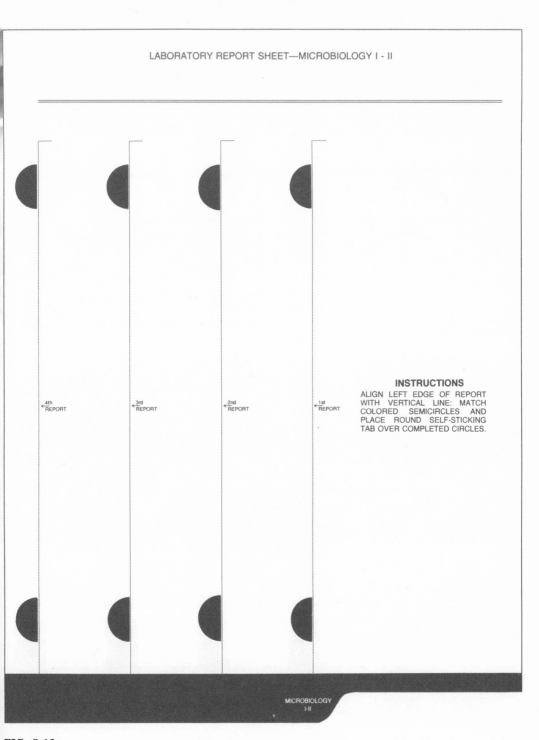

FIG. 5-12
Attachment sheet with provisions for affixing a maximum of four
microbiology reports.

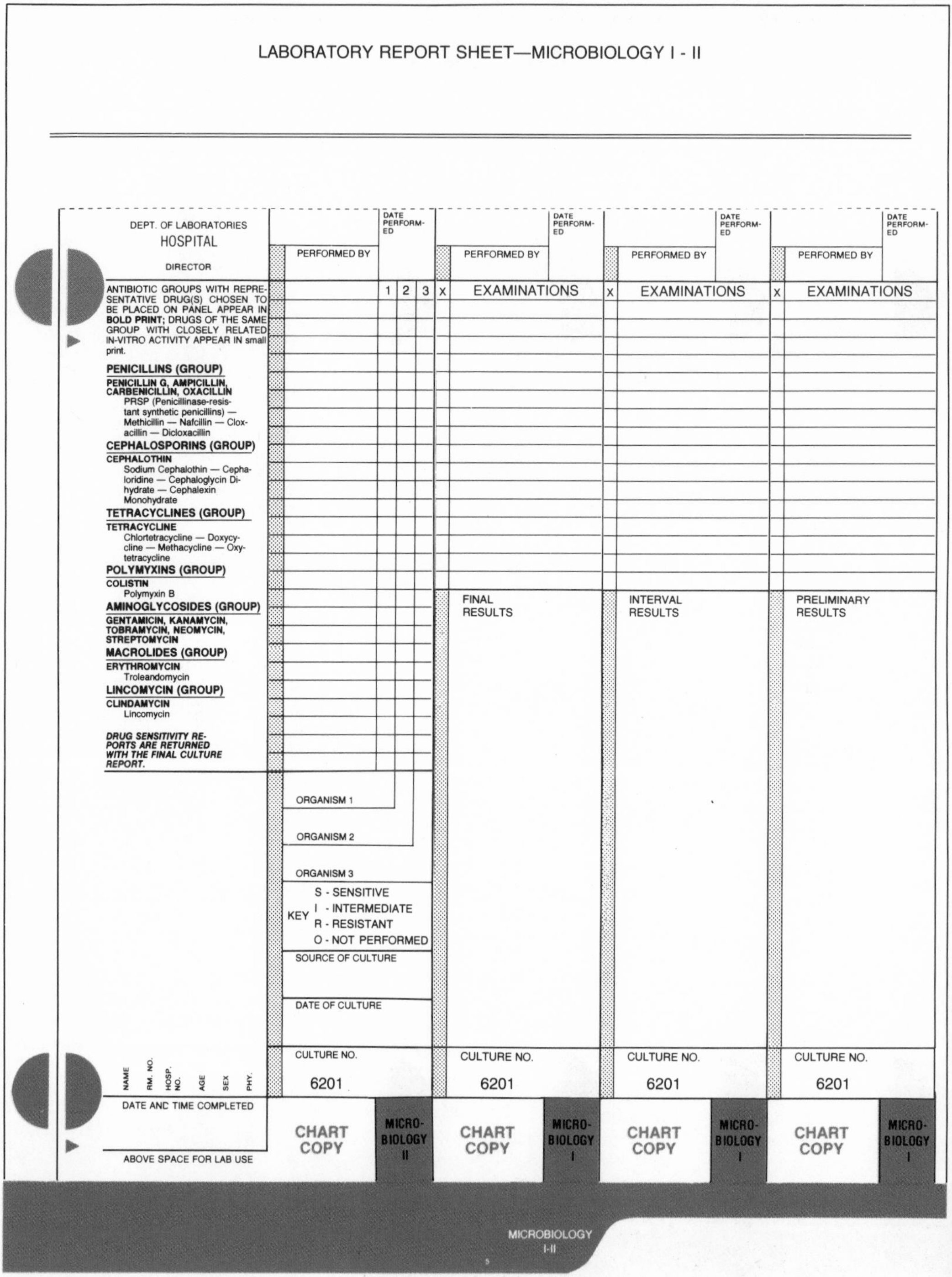
LABORATORY REPORT SHEET—MICROBIOLOGY I - II

DEPT. OF LABORATORIES
HOSPITAL
DIRECTOR

ANTIBIOTIC GROUPS WITH REPRESENTATIVE DRUG(S) CHOSEN TO BE PLACED ON PANEL APPEAR IN **BOLD PRINT;** DRUGS OF THE SAME GROUP WITH CLOSELY RELATED IN-VITRO ACTIVITY APPEAR IN small print.

PENICILLINS (GROUP)
PENICILLIN G, AMPICILLIN, CARBENICILLIN, OXACILLIN
PRSP (Penicillinase-resistant synthetic penicillins) — Methicillin — Nafcillin — Cloxacillin — Dicloxacillin

CEPHALOSPORINS (GROUP)
CEPHALOTHIN
Sodium Cephalothin — Cephaloridine — Cephaloglycin Dihydrate — Cephalexin Monohydrate

TETRACYCLINES (GROUP)
TETRACYCLINE
Chlortetracycline — Doxycycline — Methacycline — Oxytetracycline

POLYMYXINS (GROUP)
COLISTIN
Polymyxin B

AMINOGLYCOSIDES (GROUP)
GENTAMICIN, KANAMYCIN, TOBRAMYCIN, NEOMYCIN, STREPTOMYCIN

MACROLIDES (GROUP)
ERYTHROMYCIN
Troleandomycin

LINCOMYCIN (GROUP)
CLINDAMYCIN
Lincomycin

DRUG SENSITIVITY REPORTS ARE RETURNED WITH THE FINAL CULTURE REPORT.

PERFORMED BY | DATE PERFORMED
1 2 3
ORGANISM 1
ORGANISM 2
ORGANISM 3
KEY S - SENSITIVE
I - INTERMEDIATE
R - RESISTANT
O - NOT PERFORMED
SOURCE OF CULTURE
DATE OF CULTURE
CULTURE NO.
6201

NAME RM. NO. HOSP. NO. AGE SEX PHY.
DATE AND TIME COMPLETED
ABOVE SPACE FOR LAB USE

CHART COPY | MICRO-BIOLOGY II

PERFORMED BY | DATE PERFORMED
X EXAMINATIONS
FINAL RESULTS
CULTURE NO.
6201
CHART COPY | MICRO-BIOLOGY I

PERFORMED BY | DATE PERFORMED
X EXAMINATIONS
INTERVAL RESULTS
CULTURE NO.
6201
CHART COPY | MICRO-BIOLOGY I

PERFORMED BY | DATE PERFORMED
X EXAMINATIONS
PRELIMINARY RESULTS
CULTURE NO.
6201
CHART COPY | MICRO-BIOLOGY I

MICROBIOLOGY I-II

FIG. 5-13
Attachment of a maximum of four microbiology reports to any one attachment sheet.

LABORATORY REPORT SHEET—BLOOD BANK

DEPT. OF LABORATORIES HOSPITAL DIRECTOR		DATE PERFORM-ED			DATE PERFORM-ED			DATE PERFORM-ED			DATE PERFORM-ED
	PERFORMED BY			PERFORMED BY			PERFORMED BY			PERFORMED BY	
SUBMITTED BY	X	TEST	RESULT	X	TEST	RESULT	X	TEST	RESULT	X	TEST	RESULT
DATE AND TIME SUBMITTED												

REQUEST SPECIFICATIONS
TIME

☐ ROUTINE
☐ TODAY
☐ STAT
☐ SPECIFIC TIME

CONDITIONS

☐ PREADMISSION
☐ ADMISSION
☐ PREOP ___ DATE OF SURGERY

PATIENT CATEGORY

☐ INPATIENT
☐ OUTPATIENT
☐ EMERGENCY ROOM
☐ OTHER

NAME & CODE
SPECIAL INSTRUCTIONS

ATTENTION–*PLEASE COMPLETE ALL ITEMS ABOVE*

TRANSFUSION SERVICES SUBMIT SEPARATE REQUEST FOR EACH UNIT ORDERED	TRANSFUSION SERVICES SUBMIT SEPARATE REQUEST FOR EACH UNIT ORDERED	TRANSFUSION SERVICES SUBMIT SEPARATE REQUEST FOR EACH UNIT ORDERED	TRANSFUSION SERVICES SUBMIT SEPARATE REQUEST FOR EACH UNIT ORDERED
OTHER	OTHER	OTHER	OTHER

CROSSMATCH RESULTS, BLOOD (×4)

DONOR NUMBER			DONOR NUMBER			DONOR NUMBER			DONOR NUMBER		
BLOOD TYPE	DONOR	PATIENT	BLOOD TYPE	DONOR	PATIENT	BLOOD TYPE	DONOR	PATIENT	BLOOD TYPE	DONOR	PATIENT
ABO			ABO			ABO			ABO		
Rho (D)			Rho (D)			Rho (D)			Rho (D)		
CROSS-MATCH	MAJOR		CROSS-MATCH	MAJOR		CROSS-MATCH	MAJOR		CROSS-MATCH	MAJOR	
SALINE			SALINE			SALINE			SALINE		
ALB.			ALB.			ALB.			ALB.		
COOMBS			COOMBS			COOMBS			COOMBS		

RHoGAM STUDIES (×4)

RhoGAM NUMBER		RhoGAM NUMBER		RhoGAM NUMBER		RhoGAM NUMBER	
BABY Rho	POS. ☐ NEG. ☐	BABY Rho	POS. ☐ NEG. ☐	BABY Rho	POS. ☐ NEG. ☐	BABY Rho	POS. ☐ NEG. ☐
MOTHER Rho	POS. ☐ NEG. ☐	MOTHER Rho	POS. ☐ NEG. ☐	MOTHER Rho	POS. ☐ NEG. ☐	MOTHER Rho	POS. ☐ NEG. ☐
MOTHER COOMBS	POS. ☐ NEG. ☐	MOTHER COOMBS	POS. ☐ NEG. ☐	MOTHER COOMBS	POS. ☐ NEG. ☐	MOTHER COOMBS	POS. ☐ NEG. ☐
X-MATCH COMPAT.	YES ☐ NO ☐	X-MATCH COMPAT.	YES ☐ NO ☐	X-MATCH COMPAT.	YES ☐ NO ☐	X-MATCH COMPAT.	YES ☐ NO ☐
RhoGAM AVAIL.	YES ☐ NO ☐	RhoGAM AVAIL.	YES ☐ NO ☐	RhoGAM AVAIL.	YES ☐ NO ☐	RhoGAM AVAIL.	YES ☐ NO ☐
COMMENTS		COMMENTS		COMMENTS		COMMENTS	

NAME RM. NO. HOSP. NO. AGE SEX PHY.

DATE AND TIME COMPLETED

ABOVE SPACE FOR LAB USE

CHART COPY	BLOOD BANK	CHART COPY	BLOOD BANK	CHART COPY	BLOOD BANK	CHART COPY	BLOOD BANK

BLOOD BANK

FIG. 5-14

Attachment of a maximum of four blood bank reports to any one attachment sheet.

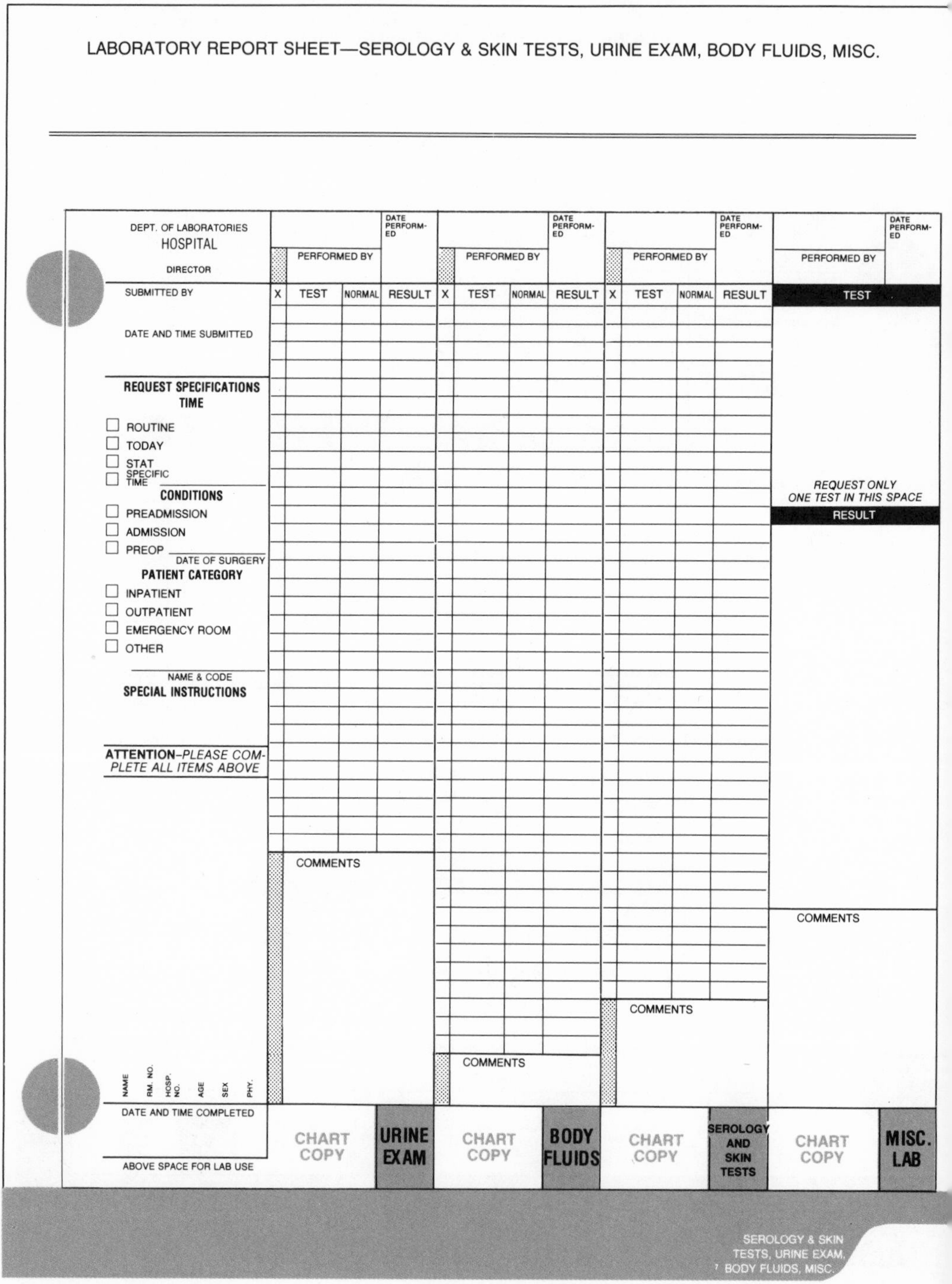

LABORATORY REPORT SHEET—SEROLOGY & SKIN TESTS, URINE EXAM, BODY FLUIDS, MISC.

DEPT. OF LABORATORIES HOSPITAL DIRECTOR			DATE PERFORM-ED			DATE PERFORM-ED			DATE PERFORM-ED		DATE PERFORM-ED
		PERFORMED BY			PERFORMED BY			PERFORMED BY		PERFORMED BY	
SUBMITTED BY	X	TEST	NORMAL	RESULT	X	TEST	NORMAL	RESULT	X	TEST	NORMAL	RESULT	TEST

DATE AND TIME SUBMITTED

REQUEST SPECIFICATIONS
TIME
☐ ROUTINE
☐ TODAY
☐ STAT
☐ SPECIFIC TIME
CONDITIONS
☐ PREADMISSION
☐ ADMISSION
☐ PREOP _____ DATE OF SURGERY
PATIENT CATEGORY
☐ INPATIENT
☐ OUTPATIENT
☐ EMERGENCY ROOM
☐ OTHER

NAME & CODE
SPECIAL INSTRUCTIONS

ATTENTION–*PLEASE COMPLETE ALL ITEMS ABOVE*

REQUEST ONLY ONE TEST IN THIS SPACE
RESULT

COMMENTS

COMMENTS

COMMENTS

COMMENTS

NAME RM. NO. HOSP. NO. AGE SEX PHY.

DATE AND TIME COMPLETED

ABOVE SPACE FOR LAB USE

CHART COPY | URINE EXAM | CHART COPY | BODY FLUIDS | CHART COPY | SEROLOGY AND SKIN TESTS | CHART COPY | MISC. LAB

SEROLOGY & SKIN TESTS, URINE EXAM, BODY FLUIDS, MISC.

FIG. 5-15
Attachment of a maximum of four different report forms to any one attachment sheet.

LABORATORY REPORT SHEET—SPECIAL REPORT

3rd REPORT ↑

2nd REPORT ↑

1st REPORT ↑

INSTRUCTIONS

ALIGN TOP EDGE OF REPORT WITH HORIZONTAL LINE; MATCH BLACK SEMICIRCLES AND PLACE ROUND SELF-STICKING TAB OVER COMPLETED CIRCLES.

SPECIAL
REPORT
8

FIG. 5-16
Attachment sheet for special reports with provisions for attachment from bottom to top.

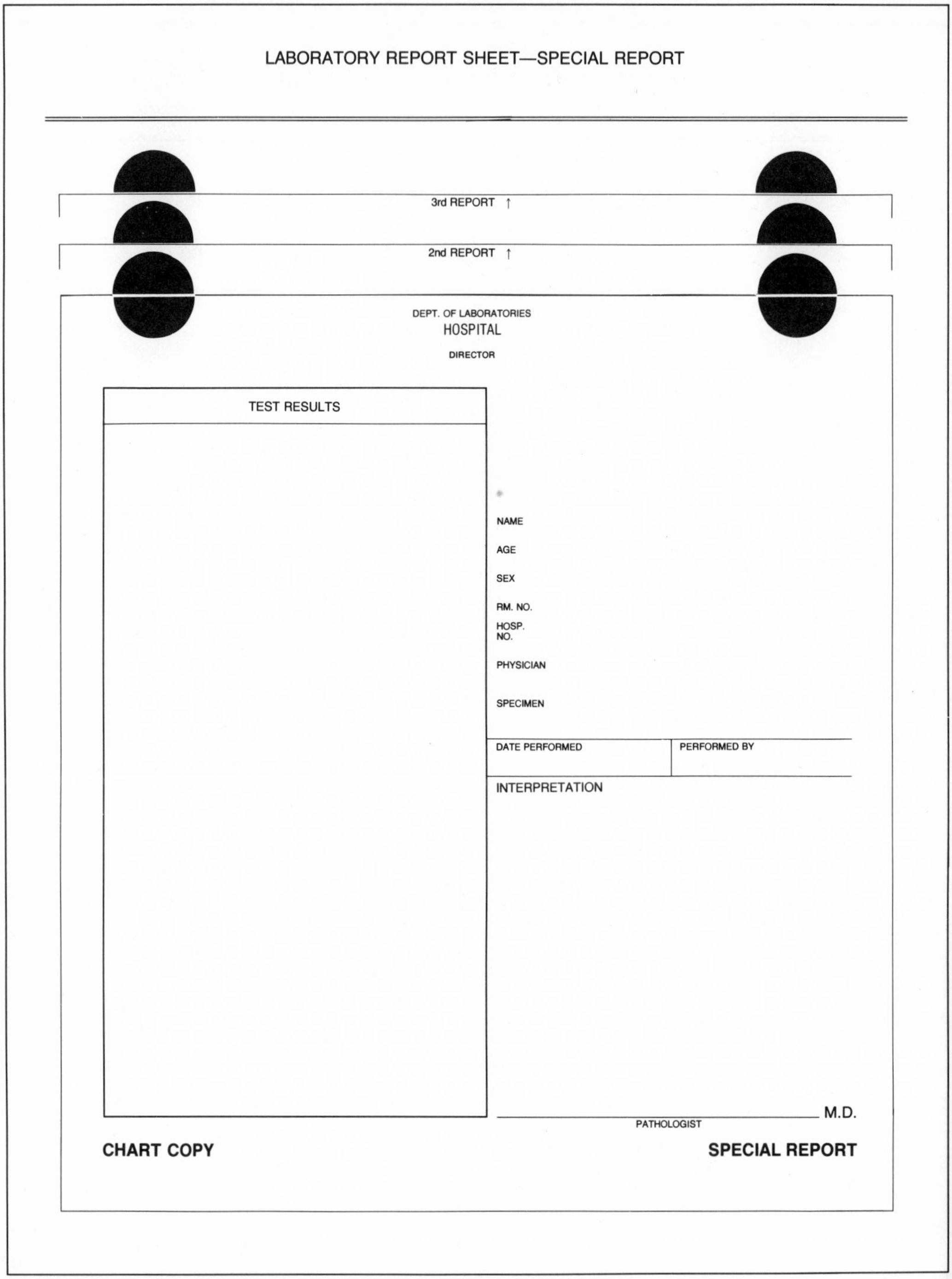

LABORATORY REPORT SHEET—SPECIAL REPORT

3rd REPORT ↑

2nd REPORT ↑

DEPT. OF LABORATORIES
HOSPITAL
DIRECTOR

TEST RESULTS

NAME

AGE

SEX

RM. NO.

HOSP.
NO.

PHYSICIAN

SPECIMEN

DATE PERFORMED	PERFORMED BY

INTERPRETATION

_____ M.D.
PATHOLOGIST

CHART COPY

SPECIAL REPORT

FIG. 5-17

7½ by 8½ inch "special report" that permits entry of a large number of test results and provides adequate space for any necessary interpretation.

LABORATORY REPORT SHEET—SPECIAL REPORT

3rd REPORT ↑

2nd REPORT ↑

DEPT. OF LABORATORIES
HOSPITAL

ELECTROPHORETOGRAM

NAME

AGE

SEX

RM. NO.

HOSP.
NO.

PHYSICIAN

PROTEIN ELECTROPHORESIS	NORMAL	RESULT
TOTAL PROTEIN	6.2-8.5 Gm./dl.	Gm./dl.
ALBUMIN	52 - 66% TOT.	% TOT.
ALPHA 1 GLOBULIN	2.0 - 6.0% TOT.	% TOT.
ALPHA 2 GLOBULIN	6.5 - 16.5% TOT.	% TOT.
BETA GLOBULIN	7.5 - 20% TOT.	% TOT.
GAMMA GLOBULIN	10 - 21% TOT.	% TOT.
ALB./GLOBULIN RATIO	1.1 - 2.2	

LDH ISOENZYMES	NORMAL (INTERNATIONAL NOMENCLATURE)	RESULT
TOTAL LDH	40 - 145 mU./ml.	mU./ml.
FRACTION 1 (LDH$_1$)	20 - 34% TOT.	% TOT.
FRACTION 2 (LDH$_2$)	29 - 41% TOT.	% TOT.
FRACTION 3 (LDH$_3$)	16 - 25% TOT.	% TOT.
FRACTION 4 (LDH$_4$)	4.0 - 12% TOT.	% TOT.
FRACTION 5 (LDH$_5$)	7.0 - 15% TOT.	% TOT.

DATE PERFORMED   PERFORMED BY

INTERPRETATION

_____ M.D.
PATHOLOGIST

CHART COPY   **SPECIAL REPORT**

FIG. 5-18

"Special report" with modification of "test results" section for
facilitating particularly unique reports.

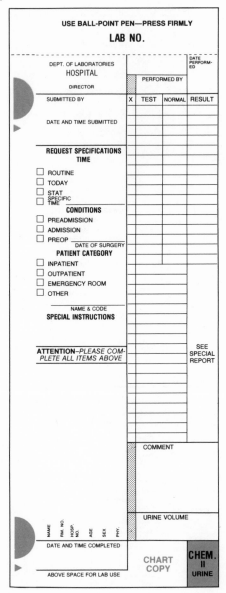

FIG. 5-19

Method for alerting the person making the request that results will be returned on a "special report" form.

efforts is greatly assisted by clear and accurate communication and an understanding and mutual respect for each department's contributions to the comfort and well-being of the patient.

Other hospital personnel

All laboratory workers should recognize the assistance they are rendered by a large number of hospital personnel. The support provided by housekeeping, dietary, maintenance, and purchasing employees, to mention only a few, is worthy of a show of appreciation by daily cordial relations.

Sales representatives

Contacts and meetings with persons from outside the hospital occur almost daily in the laboratory. Of these, contacts with salesmen occur perhaps most frequently. Information gleaned from such meetings contributes to the laboratory worker's general awareness of new products; this is deemed sufficient reason for seeing all vendors. Interviews should be arranged promptly out of courtesy and consideration for the appointment and travel schedules of salespersons. The reputation of the department as a businesslike and well-managed organization can be enhanced by the manner in which these meetings are conducted. Every effort should be made to be courteous and attentive and to impart a professional image.

REQUEST/ REPORT FORMS

The mission of the hospital laboratory is to assist the physician in the delivery of patient care by providing timely and accurate services. This implies a request/report system that is clearly understood by all participants. Of major importance to this formidable communications task are the forms with which it is conducted.

Multiple-part forms which provide both requests and

reports, represent one of the best formats for a manual hospital laboratory communications system. When properly designed, they minimize handwriting, permit convenient handling, provide standardized instructions, and generate inexpensive copies.

The forms must be of such size to be accommodated by 8½ times 11 inch sheets to which the original is customarily attached (chart). Furthermore, forms must be easy to transport, handle, sort, and store. For these and other reasons, the forms we have developed are 3 by 9¼ inches and always vertically positioned (Fig. 5-1).

Each laboratory within the department has its own form(s). They are identified by name (Microbiology, Chemistry, Hematology, etc.) and have a sufficient number of parts to permit the necessary distribution. They are manufactured to provide clear copies (carbon paper) and easy detachment (perforations at one end). The first copy (chart) is identified by color; the remaining copies are not. The color coding is for ease of identification and to facilitate chart attachment. The names of the facility and its director (a legal requirement in some states) are also included (Fig. 5-2).

Each form is divided lengthwise in half, one side for request information and the other for results. Because of their equal width, either column could accommodate these information categories. For the remainder of this presentation we will assume that the request information occupies the left column and the report data the right.

The information on the request side (left column) is arranged so that it always appears in the same descending order. This consistency serves to standardize the form and to facilitate its correct usage. When coupled with meaningful request information, this aids in securing a confident response. This information can be varied at the discretion of each facility but in all instances should permit a timely flow of services.

We recommend that the column include identification of the person who completed the request and the time of its delivery. We also suggest *time specifications* for clearly denoting the promptness with which results are needed, *conditions specifications* for indicating the circumstances bearing on the specimen collection, and *patient categories* for compiling laboratory statistical data. Additional spaces are allotted for comments deemed necessary for reliable test performance (special instructions) and *patient identification*. Finally, the time of test completion is inserted. This appears at the bottom of the column only because of the time clock mechanism that exists at the facility where these forms were conceived (Fig. 5-3).

The result column includes a list of test procedures with accompanying spaces for denoting those desired, the normal values, and patient results. It provides designated areas for identification of the person who performed the test(s) and the date of completion. There are also provisions for recording any additional information or comments related to the test results (Fig. 5-4). Printing, spacing, and column headings may be easily varied and tailored to the preferences of each facility.

With respect to charting these reports, one section of the patient's hospital record (chart) is designated for their attachment. It consists of a series of 8½ by 11 inch attachment sheets that have colored tabs with numbers and the names of the report forms to be affixed. They are inserted so that each tab is clearly visible and the numbers read consecutively from left to right (Fig. 5-5). The reports are matched by name and color with the sheet and, in accordance with the instructions appearing in Fig. 5-5, are attached in the time sequence of the test performance.

This placement of the reports results in rapid identification, alignment, and recognition of the date of test performance (Fig. 5-6). It segregates the reports by laboratory and provides convenient positioning by which the physician can rapidly compare test results. Any desire to change direction of the mounting requires only a reversal of request/report form columns and the attachment sheet lines.

This system has inconsistencies, but they are few and small. On one microbiology form a large space is provided in the right column for the lengthy reports often generated by these laboratories. Additional minor variations result from provisions for identifying specimen source and culture number. A second microbiology form (drug susceptibility studies) is generated internally by the microbiology laboratory and incorporates special left and right column contents (Fig. 5-7). Because of reporting requirements unique to blood banks, a minor variation occurs in the right column of these forms (Fig. 5-8).

Semicircles or other matching configurations (Fig. 5-9) provide the rapid and precise alignment so essential to this system of mounting. In the case of the semicircles, placement of round self-adhesive tabs over the now-completed circle provides neat and secure final attachment at a large cost reduction when compared with peel strips, which are expensive and do not provide the critical tolerance for precise alignment (see Figs. 5-6 and 5-10). With some variations to be explained later, up to nine reports may be affixed to one attachment sheet (Fig. 5-10).

Finally, a very convenient and inexpensive specimen identification system may be generated using prenumbered forms with gummed specimen container labels that are identically numbered and attached to the back of the form during the printing and manufacturing process (Fig. 5-11).

The remaining variations concern the charting phase of the system. Because of the modifications mentioned earlier, a maximum of only four microbiology and blood bank forms may be affixed to any one attachment sheet (Figs. 5-

12 to 5-14). Also, when different reports are affixed, only four can be accommodated (see Fig. 5-15).

A significant number of test results cannot be satisfactorily reported in the space provided by these forms. They include group tests, sophisticated procedures requiring interpretive remarks, and tests needing graphic evidence in support of conclusions (electrophoretograms, etc.). For these reasons, special forms are necessary for a complete hospital laboratory reporting system.

Fig. 5-5 displays the ease with which such reports can be incorporated into this system. Tab 8 in this figure signifies the location of the attachment sheet on which these reports are mounted and is the same size as all others, but with a change in format so that the lines and semicircles are arranged horizontally. The attachment of reports is thus made from bottom to top rather than right to left (Fig. 5-16).

The special report forms are multiple-part and measure 7½ by 8½ inches. Three reports are accommodated by each attachment sheet. Because of their size, they permit entry of a large number of test results with additional space for interpretation (Fig. 5-17). The "test results" section of the forms may be designed for reporting specific laboratory procedures (Fig. 5-18).

These special forms serve solely for reporting and are generated within the laboratory after receipt of one of the previously described request/report forms. The insertion of an appropriate comment in the test result column of these forms alerts the person making the request that the results will be returned on a "special report" (Fig. 5-19).

The request/report forms presented have many advantages. These include (1) consistent arrangement of information, which promotes correct usage; (2) ease with which modifications can be made to suit personal preferences; (3) color coding for ease of identification and chart attachment; (4) vertical overlapping chart attachment, which

73

permits up to nine reports per attachment sheet and facilitates rapid comparison of test results; (5) accommodations for total laboratory reporting with minimal variation in format; and (6) *rapid, inexpensive, and precise alignment and attachment of reports provided at large cost savings when compared with peel strip devices.*

6

PERSONNEL RELATIONS AND DEVELOPMENT

Personnel relations are efforts to assist an organization by enhancing the self-esteem and satisfaction of its members. More specifically, personnel relations involve fair employment practices, equitable dealings, and the opportunity for productive long-term tenure.

We must appreciate at the outset that self-preservation is the most fundamental human instinct, and all conduct is a response or reaction perceived to provide the greatest assurance of well-being. The components of this survival instinct are often stated as basic needs (food, clothing, shelter), safety and security, achievement, self-esteem, and self-actualization. In clearer terms, these may be restated as pay, challenge, and recognition. With some variations in relative importance from one person to another, they are common to all laboratory workers.

In attempting to apply this fundamental concept to the hospital laboratory, we are assuming that satisfaction of these needs depends on confident and competent job performance. An understanding of the how, why, when, and where of the job gives each employee self-assurance and the satisfaction of daily personal achievement. To assist workers to gain this satisfaction a clear definition of duties and responsibilities is necessary. Too often, unsatisfactory job performance is judged solely as the fault of the employee rather than as a result of weaknesses in the chain of command. These weaknesses often begin at the top with failure to generate and/or communicate information and instructions required for satisfactory compliance with organizational standards.

In addition to the contributions of well-conceived and clearly defined job responsibilities, sustained employee satisfaction is further aided by an environment that encourages and provides the opportunity to constantly grow and develop. The usual and customary pay increases may help avoid total insurrection, but add little to generating and holding genuine interest and enthusiasm. If employees have a continuing challenge and the opportunity to contribute, morale is increased and there is a greater chance for success of the hospital laboratory and the personal gratification of all its members.

SALARIES

In a well-planned and well-organized hospital laboratory, all job positions are defined and documented, requirements for filling each position are established, and all positions are indicated on a thoughtfully structured table of organization. On this basis, each position may be rated by the degree of difficulty and responsibility and assigned payment relative to all other jobs in the organization. This fundamental operational concept simply and objectively identifies the need for certain types of performance, the background and experience necessary to render this performance, and financial compensation that is competitive and commensurate with the degree of responsibility.

The common practice of basing hospital laboratory pay rates solely on education and certification is unfair and causes both immediate and long-term problems. How can different levels of education be used to justify sizable differences in pay among employees who all are competently performing identical jobs? This unorthodox practice has too long existed in hospital laboratories as the result of faulty assessments by directors and administrators and undue influence by special interest groups.

Pay increases are granted at the times indicated by hospital policy. They are best awarded as a percentage of base pay and, with few exceptions, should be the same for each employee. Variations based on arbitrary (and usually biased) judgments of minor differences in the quality of efforts is an exercise in foolish authoritarianism that inevitably breeds undesirable secretiveness, dissension, and discord. It is our judgment that only sizable deviations permit confident and objective assessments. If the work is obviously outstanding, promotion must be considered; if clearly unacceptable, dismissal is justified. If neither—by far the most common experience—the percentage should remain the same for all employees.

Contrary to more generally accepted practices, which attempt to identify subtle variations in performance and reward these with differing pay increases, the preceding recommendations are based on a strong belief that sufficiently accurate measurements of productivity and value do not exist to permit reliable judgments of the variations so often only suspected. Also, when infrequent extreme variations from the usual are observed, they may be rewarded or eliminated as previously indicated to the satisfaction and approval of all members of the organization.

PERSONNEL SELECTION

Good managers invariably hold that all team positions are important and any weakness has the potential for damaging the entire effort. Personnel selection thus becomes a critical operational responsibility since each new employee's abilities must match the requirements of the job. The single challenge of the organization should be to develop that person's capabilities beyond those certain at the time of employment.

The concept of personnel selection implies that a position exists and requirements for employment are known. Too often, however, many of the commonly recommended methods of assessing prospective employees are difficult and unrealistic. How, other than subjectively, are evaluations made of a person's ethics, ambition, ability to get along with others, reaction to stress, etc.? For that matter, of what value are recommendations from selected prior associates? In the last analysis, it is basically a decision of how closely the applicant's credentials match with carefully selected and quantifiable job duties.

The fact that a person takes part in a job interview does not mean that he or she will decide to fill the position. The best applicants expect the organization to be a place where people are recognized and encouraged, all jobs are important, personnel practices are fair, and management is consistent and progressive. The projection of this image requires frank and open admission of both the strengths and weaknesses of the organization and the applicant's potential role in assisting the total effort. During the interview the table of organization, job description, basic organizational philosophy, and general conditions of employment should be discussed. Hopefully, this honest exchange will result in a clearly understood and desirable matching of both parties' objectives and a mutually satisfactory professional relationship.

PERSONNEL
EVALUATION

Despite the espoused benefits of personnel evaluations, serious weaknesses exist in most methods. The weaknesses pertain largely to the questionable relevance of the assessment factors generally employed and the finely divided scales by which they are quantitated. Attendance and punctuality can be methodically and accurately measured. Attitudes, alertness, and resourcefulness defy fair and objective appraisals. When these difficulties are coupled with the varying perceptions of those persons conducting the evaluations, the effort provides questionable data by which an employee can be judged.

We are not arguing against periodic review of performance. However, we are concerned about the fairness and the degree to which the time expended is proportional to the benefits derived. In our opinion most evaluation methods are excessively detailed (poor, fair, average, good, excellent, and superior). The implied accuracy cannot be supported by the crude and subjective methodology. If the number of factors and possible scores is reduced, the evaluation can retain its value and a greater consistency will be achieved with the common observation that very few performances fall above or below the wide norm.

The major value of personnel evaluations is the opportunity they afford for planned and organized review of each employee's job performance. For best results, they require not only the supervisor's assessment of the employee, but also the employee's assessment of himself. This promotes an open exchange of views on the strengths and weaknesses of the performance and, most importantly, on methods for improvement. Care must be taken to avoid the imbalance that can come from a steady unidirectional flow of judgments that is met with the employee's silent disagreement and dissatisfaction. Such an imbalance defeats the major purpose of the interview. (See Appendix B for a recommended Personnel Evaluation Form.)

PROMOTIONS

Advancement in laboratory station or rank invariably carries increased responsibility and authority. In most instances there is greater accountability for getting things done through people. This requires an ability to plan and organize and to motivate these persons. A supervisor must be able to identify basic problems and to be fair when counseling or disciplining. Recognition of these talents is not easy or always successful. The point at which an individual will lose effectiveness is difficult to predict. In the absence of viable candidates from within the organization, outside recruitment is necessary.

Hospital laboratory promotions are generally synonymous with supervisory staff selections and, because of the importance of this segment of the membership, appointments have considerable potential for either organizational improvement or harm. Personal qualities to be considered are (1) honesty, (2) ambition, (3) initiative, (4) determination, (5) enthusiasm, (6) common sense, (7) knowledge, (8) originality, (9) understanding, and (10) communicative abilities. (For explanations of these qualities, refer to the Personnel Evaluation Form in Appendix B.)

DISMISSALS

The dismissal of a hospital laboratory employee can only be construed as an organizational failure which incurs disruption and expense to the department and embarrassment and disadvantage to the employee. Because of the total unprofitability, caution must be exercised to avoid such occurrences. However, if dismissal is unavoidable, the person's employment record should be reviewed to identify the organization's errors and prevent repetition.

Astute managers recognize these potential problems quickly, and institute procedures to determine the nature of the difficulties. It may be decided that immediate dismissal is justified, but the vast majority of infractions cannot and should not be judged and dealt with so quickly and decisively. Reported incidents are investigated for fairness and accuracy. The charged person must be discreetly interviewed to determine whether the violations are deliberate defiance of fair and equitable policies, an honest challenge of poorly conceived policies, or confusion attributable to deficiencies at higher levels of authority. If it is determined that the problem is solely the fault of the accused, the person must be given fair time and opportunity to improve his or her performance. Failure to then meet standards is just reason for terminating employment. Toleration of unsatisfactory behavior beyond this point is tantamount to forfeiture of all authority.

BASIC EDUCATION CONCEPTS

The contemplation of educational programs for hospital laboratory personnel first requires a judgment of what education is. Trite and irresponsible consideration of this fundamental question portends ineffective pursuit and probable failure of both the program and its participants.

**LEVELS AND DESCRIPTIONS
OF EDUCATIONAL ATTAINMENT**

Levels of educational attainment	Descriptions of levels of educational attainment
Wisdom ↑	The use of knowledge for attaining self-satisfaction and tranquility
Knowledge ↑	The accumulation and correlation of a large number of facts common to a given field of endeavor
Fact ↑	The awareness of small amounts of assorted data the validity of which is widely accepted
Hypothesis ↑	The formulation of random theories often from poorly supported or untested data
Information	The collection of assorted ideas, opinions, observations, and reported happenings without a determination of their validity

---

81

We suggest that education is the process of learning to think for the purpose of pursuing truth. The concept of truth, although elusive, may be perceived as that upon which there is total and universal agreement. Because this criterion is rarely satisfied, truth usually can only be approximated and based on the evidence generally agreed to be best. This logic requires that all students and teachers recognize the need for frequent adjustments in their pursuits in order to accommodate the large volume of new evidence being introduced into most fields of human endeavor.

The educational process may be divided into five levels, attainment and advancement through which are dependent upon the quality of teaching and the innate perceptions, determination, and motivation of the student. The boxed material on p. 81 includes a presentation of these levels with brief explanations of each. It is intended as a guide by which the location of the "traveler" may be identified and the distance from the destination easily measured.

HOSPITAL LABORATORY TRAINING PROGRAMS

Laboratory training, in the context of this presentation, is intended to include any of the programs sponsored by the National Accrediting Agency for Clinical Laboratory Sciences (NAACLS). The decision to seek accreditation for training MT, MLT, CLA, or other students requires careful consideration of the organization's goals and resources. Educational programs carry a serious commitment and should be neither contemplated or initiated without full realization of the magnitude of the responsibility.

A few fundamental educational concepts have been presented. They are intended to serve as basic principles upon which meaningful teaching activities should rest. Worthwhile educational programs must be concerned with the pursuit of truth—distinguishing what is valid from what is not.

Those who teach should recognize the need for clearly stated fundamental principles. Teachers must provide the student with a grasp of the basics and an enthusiasm for both pursuing the many details and deducing their significance at the time they are encountered. The student must be given the means for distinguishing fact from information and stimulated to an awareness of the merits of knowledge.

Basic guidelines for the previously mentioned pro-

STUDENT PERFORMANCE OBJECTIVES

Retain—to learn and periodically recall data essential to understanding the subject

Comprehend—to learn to interpret, predict, and summarize data

Apply—to learn to use data in situations different from those in which they were taught

Synthesize—to learn to combine information into originally conceived theories

Evaluate—to learn to make choices in situations that permit alternative actions

Observe—to pay careful attention to all classroom and benchwork instruction

Respond—to learn to comply and to question

Value—to learn the relative worth of information, theory, and facts

Believe—to learn to organize a set of personal values and establish those that are persuasive and dominant

Characterize—to learn to act consistently with a set of values

Communicate—to learn to speak and write with clarity and preciseness

Relate—to learn professional conduct and the principles of organized group activity

---

grams have been established by the NAACLS and serve as useful minimal requirements. It is essential, however, that the faculty and director of a school consider lecture content and provide an organized program. *Faculty members should have a thorough understanding of their subjects, the desire to teach the subjects, and ample time for preparation and presentation.* Without these essentials, the program can only be a discredit to its sponsors, a disservice to the students, and a mockery of all meaningful educational precepts.

The basic objective of all such programs is to provide graduates with the background and enthusiasm for attaining a high level of professional competence. Graduates must be sufficiently schooled in laboratory theory and technique to permit confident growth and improvement as their experiences accumulate. Despite the differences in entry requirements and course content of the various programs, a number of objectives remain common and essential to each. (See boxed material on p. 83.) The success of any hospital laboratory training program is closely related to the achievement of these objectives.

CONTINUING EDUCATION

The longest and perhaps the most difficult phase of the learning process is the many years following exit from the formal educational environment. Hopefully, the exposure imparted the fundamental principles of reasoning, evaluating, and investigating so that continuing educational pursuits are minimally affected by detachment from these surroundings.

Too often formal schooling has been no more than long and expensive memorization courses, the contents of which are long forgotten; what remains is of little value for the challenges to be encountered. Even with ideal preparation, academic detachment, coupled with routine job duties, family responsibilities, and social involvements, tends to slowly but inevitably widen the gap between the individual's awareness and the current state of the art.

To minimize the effect of this detachment, the individual must make every effort to maintain an awareness of current thinking that may influence his or her professional endeavors. In any attempt to maintain this awareness, one must be able to distinguish those who have sound evidence to support their claims from those less inclined to use scientific methods.

Several sources and opportunities are available to those determined to continue their educational pursuits. These include many books, journals, and meetings; also inservice courses, adult education courses at colleges, etc. We again caution, however, that there are large differences in the quality of these sources; therefore, care and discretion must be exercised in their selection. Because of the many benefits of staying abreast, generous budgeting for continuing education cannot but serve the best interests of every hospital laboratory.

7

RESEARCH AND METHOD DEVELOPMENT

LABORATORY INVESTIGATIVE PROGRAMS

Although serendipity has played a major role in scientific advancement, most improvements result from a curiosity and suspicion of what might be true and a dedicated effort to establish the validity of the speculation(s). Such efforts consist of an orderly sequence of activities that include: (1) collection of all data relevant to the speculation; (2) formulation of a hypothesis as a formal expression of the speculation; (3) objective measurements of the phenomena predicted by the hypothesis; and (4) acceptance, modification, or rejection of the hypothesis based upon the fulfillment of its predictions.

An acknowledgement of the need for improvement and an understanding of the basic principles by which this is accomplished should provide ample reason for meaningful investigative efforts within every hospital laboratory. The programs must be realistic and compatible with the organization's goals and expertise and, therefore, may range from formal and full-time duties to simply encouraging all personnel to be alert to operational weaknesses and seek methods of improvement.

Such programs require only recognition of the importance of new ideas to every organization and the potential of all members for making such contributions. These same persons should also be made to realize that every improvement, large or small, is significant and not necessarily dependent on education or organizational rank, but rather on close observation, curiosity, and a determination to make things better.

To maintain orderliness, all investigative efforts must be well supported by statements giving reasons for the projects, the methods by which they will be conducted, and the expected benefits. The proposals are channeled in accordance with the department's table of organization and require final approval by the director. A well-conducted program, in addition to enhancing operational efficiencies and product quality, creates an enthusiasm for constant achievement and a pride of membership in a commitment to excellence.

METHOD EVALUATION AND SELECTION

A basic operational requirement of the hospital laboratory is a well-conceived program for evaluating and selecting test methods. Parameters must be assessed to best determine the overall quality and reliability of any given procedure. Only in this manner can consistent and objective evaluation be conducted, and poor and inept selections eliminated. When carefully performed and documented, these evaluation criteria provide the analyst with an awareness of both the strengths and weaknesses of each test and provide rigid standards for comparing alternative methodology. The following assessment factors are considered to be of greatest importance in making these selections.

Precision

Precision may be defined as the extent to which measurements are repeated. The assessment is made by replicate analyses of a biological control containing stable and measurable amounts of the appropriate constituent(s) and expressed as the magnitude of error inherent in the method.

87

Control specimen requirements are easily satisfied by biological material that has been frozen, lyophilized, or otherwise preserved to stabilize the constituent concentration. Previously assayed controls are not needed and only add unnecessary expense.

After selection of the control, a minimum of twenty replicate assays are performed and stated as:

(1) Standard deviation (SD) $= \sqrt{\dfrac{\Sigma(x - \bar{x})^2}{n - 1}}$ or

(2) Coefficient of variation $= \dfrac{\text{SD}}{\bar{x}} \times 100\%$

where
x = observed individual values
$\bar{x}$ = the mean of the observed values
n = the total number of analyses

Accuracy

Accuracy may be defined as the extent to which measurements approach the "true" quantity of the constituent being analyzed; measurements must be conducted on a reference material having a known composition and concentration. The accuracy evaluation may be performed by recovery experiments, such as the addition of measured amounts of the standard to a biological specimen that has been previously assayed for the same constituent represented by the standard. Although measurements of this type are not entirely satisfactory, they do provide some information concerning the losses incurred during the analysis. The known value is plotted against the assayed value. The assay is more accurate the closer such slope is to unity (Fig. 7-1).

A number of such references (standards) may be purchased or prepared by the analyst, but limited availability continues to seriously hamper accuracy assessments in

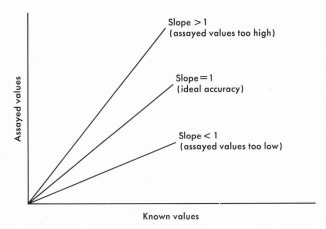

FIG. 7-1
Accuracy evaluation.

many areas of the hospital laboratory. In the absence of standards, biological controls often serve as the only reference material available to the analyst. The constituent concentration of these controls is most often stated as a mean value of replicate analyses performed by the manufacturer.

Sensitivity

Sensitivity may be defined as either (1) the extent to which the minimum amount of constituent can be measured or (2) the reliability of a test to be positive in the presence of the disease it was designed to detect. The correct use of the term is contingent upon whether one refers to the measurement of a given constituent or the ability of a test to *confirm* a suspected disease. The former can be made only by appropriate measurements while the latter is best satisfied by a literature search or original investigation.

Specificity

Specificity may be defined as either (1) the extent to which measurements are those of a single constituent (it is a measure of biochemical interference) or (2) the reliability of a test to be negative in the absence of the disease it was designed to detect.

The appropriate use of either of these definitions is determined by whether one is speaking of (1) the interference by other biochemical moieties for a given test procedure when measuring a specific constituent or (2) the ability with which the procedure can accurately *exclude* a suspected disease process. In either case, original investigation or a methodical literature search for the experience of others with the many factors that can spuriously affect laboratory test results is required. One compilation of such data may be found in the April 1975 issue of *Clinical Chemistry*.*

---

*Vol. 21, no. 5, American Association of Clinical Chemists Inc., P. O. Box 5218, Winston Salem, N.C. 27103.

8

QUALITY CONTROL

GENERAL
PRINCIPLES

Quality control is a program for assuring reliability. Such
programs vary with the product, available expertise, and
the limitations of resources. In the case of hospital laboratories, the product is test data; standards of quality include
timeliness of performance, accuracy of results, and effectiveness of communication.

Meaningful quality control in the hospital laboratory
requires an appreciation of the scope of the program.
Many of the activities occur away from the laboratory
bench so that solely monitoring test measurements does not
suffice. Fig. 8-1 diagrams these basic activities. They are
divided into analytical and nonanalytical functions and are
discussed below.

It is easy to overlook the details of such a program and
suffer from this neglect. The sheer number of duties tends
to discourage one from perceiving their importance and
the attention demanded by each. Discussion of nonanalytical control includes a number of activities that
can be considered mundane and obvious. However,
we believe that appreciating and understanding their importance far outweighs any risk of offending or boring
the reader.

91

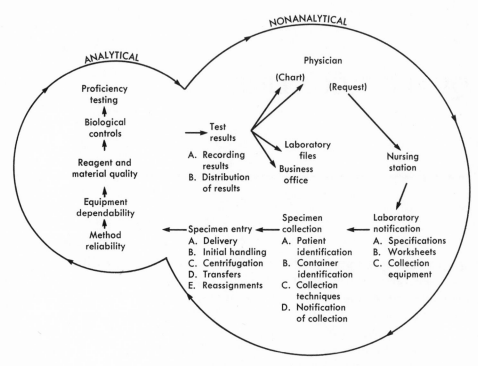

FIG. 8-1
Hospital laboratory quality control functions.

NONANALYTI-CAL QUALITY CONTROL FUNCTIONS
Physician requests

Reliable communication of the physician's needs is of such great importance to the effective delivery of laboratory services that major efforts must be extended to assure correct conduct. Unless all requests are stated clearly, serious misunderstandings and mistakes can easily occur.

A major requirement for reducing these damaging communication errors is carefully designed and standardized request/report forms. (See Request/Report Forms, Chapter 5.) Directions for using them are best supplied by instruction manuals. Their correct use is implemented by periodic in-service programs with nursing service and by giving immediate explanations to all persons who deviate from prescribed procedure.

The entire system for providing hospital laboratory services is triggered at the moment of laboratory notification. Request form information is critical to the effectiveness of this response. These instructions (specifications) must be explicit. They must constantly and consistently designate the promptness with which test results are needed (time specifications—"routine," "stat," etc.) and the patient's circumstances at the time of specimen collection (conditions specifications—"pre-op," "preadmission," etc.). Patient category specifications ("in-patient," "out-patient," etc.) facilitate subsequent compilation of laboratory statistics. (See Request/Report Forms, Chapter 5.)

Because of their major impact on services, each time specification must reliably indicate how quickly the laboratory will respond. This time is generally expressed as a maximum interval and, whether by design or bad habit, it is almost always totally used! It is important that the intervals are not so casually employed as to encourage delays in service. They should, rather, serve only as a time frame during any portion of which a response is initiated and completed in accordance with the most efficient utilization of personnel and resources. Suggested time specifications with responses to be met or exceeded are shown in boxed material below.

Routine—response and test results *within* 24 hours. May take longer for some procedures (cultures, reassignments, etc.)

Today—response and test results *within* 8 hours

Stat—response *within* 10 minutes; no delay in test performance

Specific—specimen collection *within* ± 5 minutes of time
time   designated; no delay in test performance

Worksheets

Worksheets are used most commonly for recording test results and other informative data not usually reported. However, they may be most important in helping personnel prepare for forthcoming work. A well-designed format, with patient and request entries prior to specimen arrival, enables the analyst to more effectively plan for test performance. The net effect is greater efficiency and reduced reporting time. Because worksheets are most useful when there are large numbers of scheduled procedures, they are particularly well suited to most hospital chemistry and hematology laboratories. (See Appendix B for suggested worksheet format.)

Specimen collection equipment

Prompt and efficient specimen collections can be facilitated if all equipment is maintained in a constant state of readiness. There is nothing more inopportune or untimely than a delay of services, particularly urgent services, because of a lack of necessary items.

For each item a minimum and maximum number should be determined that represents a range of quantities that is constantly maintained in each "collection basket." Stocking to maximum numbers is a logical daily responsibility of third shift personnel, while first and second shift workers may be held accountable for replenishments to at least minimum numbers on all other occasions.

Patient identification

Correct patient identification is critical to assuring reliable laboratory services. Because correct identification is of overriding importance to the patients' well-being and safety, all policies must be carefully conceived, periodically confirmed, and rigidly enforced. Laboratory workers too often display less than the caution and deliberation that such identification demands.

With some chagrin, we still recall a serious identification

error that resulted when two patients with identical names occupied the same room, and their identification numbers differed by only one digit. They were delivered of babies of the same sex on the same day by the same physician. Many readers may be reminded of similar circumstances that resulted in errors or near errors. In any event, all laboratory workers must be constantly alert to the importance of this identification process.

The customary practice in hospitals is to attach identification bands to all patients. Laboratory standards for identifying these persons demand no less than *exact* matching of *all* patient information appearing on the request with that on the bracelet. Lack of such match requires immediate correction of all discrepancies or, under certain time constraints, reliable third party assurance of the patient's identity.

Container identification

Clear and accurate container identification is necessary for several reasons: the frequency of specimen collections, multiple distributions, container transfers, delays in testing, and need for hasty retrieval. Obviously, identification must begin immediately upon specimen collection and continue through disposal.

Identification methods range from copying onto the container all patient identification information appearing on the request form to the attachment of prenumbered labels from correspondingly prenumbered request/report forms. (See Request/Report Forms, Chapter 5.) From this range of options, each laboratory must select the system that provides the most effective and reliable results.

It seems to us that once the very singular and separate function of patient identification is completed, there is no need to spend inordinate amounts of time copying (often unclearly) patient data. A much faster match is made between request form and container by the inexpensive prenumbering system mentioned above. It has been clearly established to our satisfaction that manually copying patient data consumes approximately 25 percent of total collection time for single tubes and progressively increases for multiple tubes. For a subject that has such potential for large time savings, it appears to be rather poorly addressed by many hospital laboratories.

Specimen collection techniques

Standard specimen collection techniques are found in many laboratory texts and need not be reiterated here. There is need, however, to remind laboratory personnel of the importance of these practices to every quality control program. Workers are also responsible for using correct specimen volumes and appropriate containers and additives.

Blood collections are a major function of the hospital laboratory and have a major impact on the quality of services. Their importance cannot be neglected or forgotten. Most failures at obtaining a blood sample result from hasty and poor positioning of the patient and/or phlebotomist and careless selection of the venipuncture site. If the concept of laboratory quality is expanded to include patient satisfaction and comfort, these duties assume even greater importance to the program.

Notification of specimen collection

Laboratory specimen collections frequently trigger additional services that bear significantly on the well-being of the patient. In a spirit of genuine cooperation and concern for maximum patient services, efficient notification of the nursing staff concerning these collections is highly desirable. Any one of a number of schemes can be employed, but one of the simplest and most effective is for each nursing unit to prepare a daily list of the patients on whom laboratory work has been ordered and for the laboratory to check (✔) these names promptly upon completion of the blood drawings.

Specimen entry

Alterations of specimen constituents that result from laboratory manipulation should be minimal and should occur to an equal degree in each specimen. These precautions assume particular importance when a given test is ordered in series.

Delivery of specimens

Most systems for delivering specimens to the hospital laboratory involve hand-carrying of the specimens and require standards only for assuring promptness. Alternatives exist, however, for distribution of the specimens after arrival. In indirect distribution all specimens are deposited in a designated area where they are processed (centrifuged, divided, etc.) and redistributed. Direct distribution, on the other hand, involves the straight and uninterrupted delivery of the specimen to the area in which the tests are to be performed. The personnel in these areas are held totally accountable for all subsequent proceedings. Although specimen utilization is less efficient, the latter method is preferable in most hospital laboratories because of fewer handlings, less division of responsibility, and easier identification and correction of errors and rule infractions.

Initial handling, centrifugation, and transfer of specimens

In addition to delivery and distribution efforts, the specimen entry process requires several other deliberations including methods for initial handling, centrifugation, and transfers. These are frequent daily procedures having measurable effects on test results and must be performed with care and consistency. Unless a test procedure specifically indicates otherwise, the recommendations in the box on pp. 98–99 are considered pertinent and appropriate.

INITIAL SPECIMEN HANDLING

Whole blood—keep stoppered in original container; if analysis delayed, store at 4°C–6°C.

RBCs—centrifuge blood in original container; if analysis delayed, store at 4°C–6°C.

Plasma—centrifuge blood in original container; transfer plasma immediately; if analysis delayed, store at 4°C–6°C.

Serum—allow blood to clot for 20–30 minutes in original container; gently loosen clot at top with applicator stick; centrifuge and immediately transfer serum; if analysis delayed, store at 4°C–6°C.

Urine—keep sealed in original container; if analysis delayed, store at 4°C–6°C.

Body fluids—as urine.
(CSF, etc.)

CENTRIFUGATION

General—develop and maintain preventive maintenance program for all centrifuges; periodically confirm rpm.

Balance—with regard for geometrically symmetrical arrangement, always place tubes and carriers (or shields) of equal weight, shape, and size in opposing positions of centrifuge head.

Tubes—always place tubes on rubber cushions in carriers and shields; eliminate all tubes with cracks, chips, and other flaws.

Technique—always stopper tubes; for serum or plasma separations, centrifuge for 10 minutes at 850–1000 RCF (G); always accelerate slowly and allow centrifuge to decelerate and stop at its own rate; use brake only in emergencies such as tube breakage.

SPECIMEN TRANSFERS

General—at time of transfer, always clearly and accurately identify container into which transfer is made.

Plasma—always separate immediately after centri-
and/or fuging; avoid transfer of RBCs; should
serum transfer occur, centrifuge until clear with RBC button.

Urine—always mix thoroughly by inversion immediately before transfer.

Body fluids—as urine.
(CSF, etc.)

Specimen reassignments

Reassigning specimens to a reference laboratory is considered only after the capabilities and cost of in-house performance are determined and usage is projected. Should a need for selective outside assistance be determined, a careful choice of one or more of these facilities is made.

Factors to be considered in this selection are: (1) range of available services (brochure listings); (2) quality (staff, facilities, etc.); (3) location (transportation mode); (4) turnaround time (periodic review); and (5) fee schedule (comparison with laboratories of comparable stature). In addition, hospital personnel should evaluate the brochure instructions concerning collection, packaging, and mailing of specimens and the quality of supplies provided by the reference laboratory for satisfactory compliance. Furthermore, if the outside facility fails to reference its methodology, specific inquiry is in order.

Distribution of test results

The final nonanalytical responsibilities relate to recording and distributing test results. These activities are dictated

99

largely by request/report slip format. The importance of neatness, clarity, accuracy, and completeness cannot be underestimated. In most instances, the recipients of this laboratory data include nursing station personnel (chart attachment), the hospital business office (patient bills), the attending physician (personal use), and the laboratory clerical section (department record).

Nursing station distribution

Orderly and convenient chart attachment of laboratory reports is facilitated by a clearly displayed laboratory chart section, segregation of reports by laboratory (chemistry, hematology, etc.), and a rapid and economical mounting system that permits fast identification and comparison of test results. (See Request/Report Forms, Chapter 5.) If chart attachment is a nursing station responsibility, laboratory reports should be delivered at times both convenient to allow immediate mounting and suited to the schedules of the medical staff.

Business office distribution

The business office must be notified of laboratory charges if patient bills are to be accurate. Notification schedules should be set up that are satisfactory to the two departments. The more promptly the business office is notified the less frequently patients will be billed for late charges, and there will be fewer complaints by patients who find they owe an additional amount after paying what they thought was a final bill.

One way to eliminate errors and delays in notification is to route charges immediately after specimen collection. Although this results in greater issuance of credits resulting from order changes, request errors, etc., the benefits in patient satisfaction far outweigh the small disadvantage incurred.

A separate distribution of test results to the physician provides a second source of information in the event of errors in chart attachment or oversights of data correctly affixed. If laboratory results can be promptly delivered to a central location the data can be available for physicians before they make rounds. Of no little consequence is the reduction of telephone inquiries to the laboratory effected by such distributions.

Laboratory copies of all test results are needed because data from previously done tests are frequently requested. Multiple-part request/report forms with laboratory copies filed to permit rapid retrieval meet these requirements. With regard to record keeping, in addition to the full-time efforts of hospital records personnel, our bureaucrats have once again displayed their frustrating disregard for efficiency by insisting that a portion of these activities be duplicated in the laboratory. Retention time is two years (*Federal Register,* Vol. 40, No. 41 - March 10, 1975). With these kinds of arbitrary standards by which hospital laboratories are made to operate, it is wise to caution against any additional record keeping (log books, etc.) unless the benefits firmly outweigh the disadvantages of time and transposition errors.

This is an appropriate time to comment on log books and their contributions to laboratory efforts. Too often they serve only as an unnecessary and ineffective second recording of test results. However, with an appropriate format—namely, entry sites permitting rapid recognition of a patient's preceding results—an additional means of assuring reliable services is provided.

Deviations resulting from laboratory error can be spotted immediately, thus eliminating the confusion and frustration caused by random reporting of values that differ considerably from the patient's preceding results. With log book entries permitting observation of the last results of the same test, such disparities are immediately identified and results withheld until a satisfactory explanation is determined. The amount of entry time is no greater than for customary logging. Rearrangement to permit entries by designated patient rather than consecutively is all that is required. (See Cumulative Test Records in Appendix B.)

ANALYTICAL QUALITY CONTROL FUNCTIONS

Method reliability

The reliability of laboratory test results obviously depends on the methodology employed. The range of available methods demands that, as the initial step in all analytical quality control efforts, a consistent and meaningful program of evaluation be formulated. Any neglect of this responsibility is certain to result in inept selections, the "control" of which provides few rewarding results. For a further discussion of this fundamental matter, see Chapter 7.

Equipment dependability

Equipment dependability is an essential part of every analytical quality control program and depends upon the care and maintenance provided. The quality of these efforts is contingent upon a carefully structured program of instruction and documented equipment surveillance (see Chapter 9).

Reagent and material quality

Of major importance to this phase of hospital laboratory quality control are methods for assuring test reagent and material quality. Their reliability can never be taken for granted, and they must periodically be verified to be without contamination or deterioration. The frequency of these checks is determined by the difficulties imposed, expense incurred, and availability of alternative quality assurance practices.

In the microbiology laboratory and blood bank, where testing is largely the identification of unknowns (qualitative), frequent assessments of reagent and material quality provide the only means of assuring reliable test results. In the chemistry and hematology laboratories, where testing is largely quantitation of specifically requested constituents, biological controls containing these same constituents provide an alternative one-step method for assuring total integrity of test performance. This reduces the need for frequent assessments of reagents and materials so critical in microbiology laboratories and blood banks.

This presentation is not intended to deal with the large numbers of methods for assuring reagent and material quality in the hospital laboratory. They are too numerous and unique from one area to another for any meaningful discussion here. However, in order for the laboratory worker to have a structured and organized grasp of analytical quality control, this category of activities must be recognized and its application thoughtfully deliberated.

Biological controls

The aspect of quality assurance most written about and discussed is the testing of biological controls. Satisfactory measurements of these controls provide increased confidence in the results.

Hospital laboratory measurements employ a number of scales. Qualitative measurements are concerned only with identity, i.e., presence or absence of a constituent (0 or +). Semiquantitative measurements employ a scale based on order and usually expressed as scores 0 to + + + +. Some measurements are expressed in units that become logarithmic, as when serial dilutions are made and the result is reported as the number of tubes showing the effect. Finally, measurements may be expressed as units of time or as ratios including such data as weight, volume, etc.

After selecting the test method (scales of measurement)

and appropriate controls, the laboratory worker must establish acceptable limits of unavoidable error. The methods for establishing the limits vary with the scales of measurement. Under test conditions, when control measurements fall within or outside these limits, a similar degree of error is assumed for the patient specimen and results accepted or rejected accordingly. Table 8-1 includes the usual hospital laboratory scales of measurement and the generally accepted permissible limits of unavoidable error.

As seen in Table 8-1, four scales of measurement are employed for most hospital laboratory reporting. Each of these is assigned limits of permissible error, which are determined basically by the complexity of the test methodology. Measurements of identity reject any deviation from the stated presence or absence of the given constituent. Measurements expressed as a logarithmic function are arbitrarily assigned limits of ± 1 dilution (tube). Time and ratio measurements are allowed ± 2 standard deviations (SD). Because of the more involved methodology by which permissible limits for time and ratio measurements

TABLE 8-1

Quality control measurements with permissible limits of unavoidable error

Laboratory	Usual measurement scales	Permissible limits of error
Chemistry	Ratio	± 2.0 SD
Hematology	Ratio	± 2.0 SD
Coagulation	Time	± 2.0 SD
Blood bank	Identity	None (0 or +)
Microbiology	Identity	None (0 or +)
Serology	Identity	None (0 or +)
	may be logarithmic	± 1.0 dilution
Urinalysis	Identity	None (0 or +)

are determined, more detailed treatment of this subject follows.

The relative complexity of time and ratio measurements has resulted in a number of statistical treatments for expressing the amount of permissible error. The most frequent of these is the standard deviation (SD). This is an assessment of the ability to reproduce a measurement and is calculated from a set of determinations on the same sample. Quality control purposes call for performing replicate assays ($\geq$ 20) upon multiple aliquots of the same control and calculating from the following formula:

$$SD = \sqrt{\frac{\Sigma(x - \bar{x})^2}{n - 1}}$$

Here, $(x - \bar{x})$ is the difference between the value for each measurement x and the mean of all the measurements $\bar{x}$; n is the total number of aliquots.

The permitted variation (used for subsequent assessment of daily control results) is taken as 2.0 SD. This is equivalent to saying that if a single result is drawn at random from a series of assays on the same sample, the odds are 20 to 1 that the value will not be further removed from the mean than twice the SD; or, should this value exceed the limits of 2.0 SD, there is a 95 percent chance that this has resulted from avoidable error. This equivalency can be graphically demonstrated by constructing a frequency distribution curve from the replicate control values.

The numerical value of a standard deviation for the same method can vary from one laboratory to another because of different policies and technique. This suggests that quality assurance efforts provide not only opportunity for general control over the reliability of laboratory performance, but also a means for enhancing individual proficiency. We have in mind the use of controls whose constituent concentrations are not known prior to testing (varying dilutions), and establishing the permissible limits of error (performance of the replicate assays) by the most skilled analyst(s) so that all subsequent daily testing by other workers must meet this performance.

It is well to again point out that regardless how carefully laboratory measurements are made, they are subject to degrees of unavoidable error since it is virtually impossible to duplicate day-to-day performance. These errors occurring in an otherwise controlled analysis are also expressed as random, experimental, or uncontrollable. The program is designed to determine the extent to which they occur and to reject all values exceeding permissible limits.

Excessive unavoidable error implies poor performance of reagents, equipment, analyst, or any combination of these factors. In the event of unacceptable control results one must not introduce additional factors requiring assess-

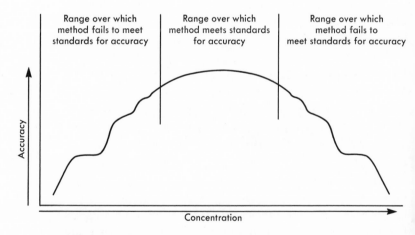

FIG. 8-2
Graphic demonstration that the constituent concentrations of the controls must fall within range over which test methods meet accuracy standards.

ment. For this reason *constituent concentrations of the control must be within the range over which the test methods meet prescribed accuracy standards.* Otherwise, investigation of failure to reproduce satisfactory control values introduces the possibility of method unreliability (Fig. 8-2).

Furthermore, if constituent concentrations are within a suitable range and *if the control efforts are solely for the purpose of assessing reproducibility of reagents, equipment, and analyst,* the recommended use of two controls at the time of each analysis or batch of analyses is poorly conceived, unduly expensive, and justified only on the dubious premise that two (or why not more?) of anything is better than one.

Control charts assist in monitoring avoidable and unavoidable errors. The usual format includes an ordinate for entering the range of values over which the control results are most likely to occur and an abscissa for recording the time intervals at which the control results are obtained. A pair of horizontal lines are included to correspond with the permitted limits (values) of unavoidable error (2.0 SD).

With each determination or batch of determinations, the analyst includes a control and plots the result. Values falling out of acceptable range are rejected as avoidable errors that must be identified and corrected. All tests belonging to this batch are repeated. In the absence of avoidable error, 95 percent of analyses should be within control values.

In addition to identifying sporadic errors that are generally caused by the analyst, control charts are helpful in determining more subtle problems manifested by trends and shifts. A *trend* occurs when control values continue to increase or decrease over consecutive days, suggesting reagent or equipment alterations. A *shift* is formed by control values that maintain a constant level on one side of the mean value line, suggesting an incorrectly prepared reagent (Fig. 8-3).

107

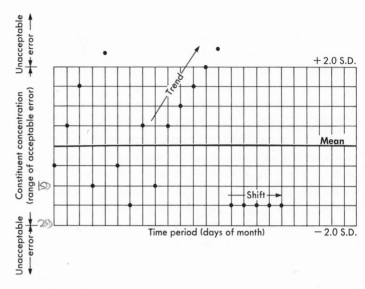

FIG. 8-3

Control chart format with examples of possible entries.

In summary, the concept of monitoring laboratory performance by the use of biological controls is valid and useful. The practice, however, must not be perceived as a singular and totally secure device. This perception can only lead to an unhealthy and ill-advised neglect of many other quality control responsibilities. Furthermore, this single aspect of the program can be disproportionately and excessively costly unless care and forethought are given to meaningful and efficient control material utilization.

Proficiency testing Widespread participation of hospital laboratories in proficiency testing programs has resulted largely from the Medicare and Clinical Laboratories Acts of 1967 and legislation recently culminated by introduction into the U.S. House of Representatives of Clinical Laboratories Improvement Act, 1978. The major thrust of this legislation is to improve the quality of laboratory services by setting forth standards of performance that must be met or exceeded.

Standards provide that each laboratory satisfactorily display an ability to make *accurate* periodic analyses of unknown samples or other material used in the proficiency program. Participation constitutes an analytical quality control activity, but for many reasons it cannot be substituted for the many daily and more important practices already cited.

In addition, standards of accuracy need more definitive analysis. Can accuracy requirements be satisfied simply by obtaining the best results possible with a method of questionable reliability; or must all results be judged by their approximation to those generated by better procedures? Toleration of results because they represent the best possible from ill-chosen methods does little to improve accuracy, the major reason for these programs!

The following general information concerns the roles of those laboratories serving specialized functions in these programs and requirements of the general participants.

A *reference laboratory* is one of recognized competence, which examines in detail proficiency testing samples or other material to authenticate identification, content, or titer. The laboratory is specially qualified by experience, interest, and accepted expertise. The analyses are done extremely carefully and are performed in replicate. The mean test result values are considered to closely approach "true" values and serve as a measurement of the accuracy of test results obtained by the participating laboratories. It is generally prescribed that there be at least four such laboratories for each commonly used method of chemical analysis and eight for morphological, serological, and microbiological identification. All samples are mailed to these facilities in advance of the general survey.

A *referee laboratory* is one of recognized competence and a general participant in the proficiency program. It uses the same time schedule and performs the examinations under the same conditions as all other general participants. The identity of these laboratories is not revealed. Their test results are used as a measure of the quality of the proficiency testing specimens and, with the reference laboratories' results, are an influencing factor in deciding the acceptable range of results.

A *participating laboratory* is enrolled in a proficiency program and adheres to testing all proficiency specimens in the *identical* manner employed for patient testing. Replicate analyses are avoided and duplicate assays are performed only when duplicate testing is a laboratory routine. Requirements for participation, frequency of specimen shipments, time allotted for returning results, and methods of grading are determined by the organization conducting the program.

9

THE CARE OF EQUIPMENT AND LABORATORY SAFETY

EQUIPMENT MAINTENANCE AND REPAIR

Carefully conceived maintenance and repair of equipment is valuable for a number of reasons. First, such a program contributes to cost savings by prolonging equipment life and diminishing expensive "down time." Second, as already indicated in Chapter 8, it constitutes an essential category of quality control. Finally, practices that reduce equipment malfunction and attending hazards must be recognized as contributing to the safety and well-being of all laboratory workers.

In general, it is advisable to hold supervisory personnel accountable for maintenance and repair of all equipment assigned to their areas. Delegation of specific maintenance duties can then be made in accordance with the degree of difficulty and recommendations of the manufacturer. Most of these functions can be performed by laboratory personnel while some are done more effectively by outside persons specializing in these services. Supervisory responsibilities should include instruction and training of personnel in the use of equipment and development of a plan for verifying and maintaining reliable performance that is conducted and documented on a scheduled basis.

The success of such a plan depends on the ease with which these duties can be identified and recorded. Too frequently the proposed methods and formats are excessively awkward and time consuming, causing inefficiencies and disconcerting loss of effectiveness.

We have devised a system that circumvents these difficulties. We use a manual that has a series of pages representing the time intervals at which specific preventive maintenance actions must be taken. The actions are identified by number, and there are spaces for the name of the instrument, action needed, and a check mark indicating that the action has been taken. In addition, each page includes prominent markers to alert personnel of less frequently required actions. In separate sections of the manual are correspondingly numbered instructions for performing each action and provisions for biannual and annual summations of equipment performance. (See Appendix B for format of Preventive Maintenance Manual.)

The manual just described is used to assure reliable daily and long-term equipment performance. However, should malfunction or breakdown occur, similarly planned action is required; *the major problem in resolving a problem is identifying the problem.* Efforts are facilitated when the workers who are most familiar with the instrument proceed, like all careful investigators, from the most to the least likely cause of the problem. They must also be able to recognize when their efforts are to no avail and assistance is required.

**SAFETY
PROGRAMS**

Laboratory safety programs are plans for preventing sickness and injury to personnel and damage or destruction of physical assets. Because of many health, monetary, legal, and environmental implications, such programs are deserving of careful attention by all laboratory workers.

Safety practices, although an important and fundamental responsibility, are too often the least deliberated and most poorly conducted. This dangerous behavior is difficult to understand, but perhaps it results because safety practices are neglected in laboratory training programs, laboratory directors and supervisors are indifferent to the problems of safety, and laboratory workers find safety programs inconvenient.

It is ill-advised to ever relegate protection of laboratory personnel to a position of secondary importance. To the contrary, the merits of cautious laboratory behavior must receive sufficient emphasis so that this behavior becomes a way of life. All personnel must be convinced of its benefits and realize that all transgressions cause a dangerous and unnecessary risk to life and limb.

Development of a meaningful and effective safety program requires a concerted effort to identify the sources of hazard and the categories of laboratory activity into which they belong. Only in this way can the program be reduced to manageable units rather than becoming an infinite number of details that defy disentanglement and thwart interest, efforts, and results. Most laboratory-incurred sickness and injury result from overcrowding, poorly maintained equipment, careless housekeeping, thoughtlessness, and inexperience. The reduction of risks within the hospital laboratory can only be considered a serious operational responsibility to which directors and supervisors must lend their full support.

The fundamental objectives of a meaningful hospital laboratory safety program are: (1) to improve safety skills and attitudes of all personnel; (2) to develop a surveillance program for promptly identifying hazards; (3) to formulate plans for promptly correcting all hazards; and (4) to coordinate laboratory safety efforts with the overall hospital safety program.

The remainder of the presentation is simply an attempt to reduce the seemingly endless number of requirements into basic categories. The many details are purposely omitted, but their insertion is easily accommodated in accordance with each laboratory's own perceptions and circumstances.

An employee health program must include:

1. Preemployment physical examinations with laboratory and radiological studies that establish fitness for laboratory employment
2. Periodic repetition of above; in most instances reassessments are made yearly, but some findings and/or working conditions dictate a shorter interval
3. Written reports of all work-related illnesses and accidents with review by director or designee
4. Employee health records for the total period of employment

A general safety program must include:

1. Orientation of new employees to department's attitudes and policies for assuring safe laboratory conduct
2. Periodic supervisory staff meetings for express purpose of discussing safety; attention is given to particular times and circumstances that lend themselves to deviation from policy (lack of supervision, excessively busy work periods, etc.)
3. Orderly housekeeping standards for both laboratory and housekeeping personnel
4. Signs indicating need for special precaution in area where posted; also, strategically placed signs indicating general need to avoid thoughtless and reckless behavior
5. Orderly storage and arrangement of supplies and working materials; insistance on adequate space
6. Policies governing eating, drinking, smoking, and safe attire within the department
7. Periodic inspections by director or designee for purpose of indicating interest and concern for program
8. Consideration of periodic programs by outside

persons with expertise in special areas of laboratory safety

9. Consideration of hiring a full- or part-time safety officer
10. Coordinated efforts with hospital for assuring isolation of communicable diseases, control of nosocomial infections, and plans for dealing with fire and disaster

A program for handling chemicals must include:

1. Prescribed containers and adequate storage space with secure shelving and proper ventilation
2. Permanent container labels with clear identification of contents; bold identification of particularly harmful chemicals
3. Policies for transporting containers, particularly if large, heavy, or filled with especially dangerous contents
4. Instructions for dispensing, transferring, and disposing of all chemicals

A program for handling biological specimens must include:

1. Instructions for collecting, transferring, storing, and disposing of all specimens
2. Policies for isolating test procedures performed on specimens suspected to contain infectious agents
3. Instructions for handwashing and the care and cleaning of work surfaces
4. Instructions for cleaning and/or disposing of specimen collection equipment

A fire prevention program must include:

1. Physical facilities and operational practices that satisfy fire code
2. Instructions for handling and storing combustibles; container labels with "flash points"
3. Instructions for operating all heat-generating equipment (gas burners, hot plates, etc.)

115

4. Well-conceived and rehearsed plans in event of fire that are closely coordinated with hospital efforts and include strategically placed and properly maintained sand buckets, fire extinguishers, and fire blankets

A first aid program must include:

1. Policies for dealing with all job-incurred injuries
2. Strategically placed and boldly identified emergency shower(s) and eye bath(s)

10

COST CONTROL

There are no hospital laboratory activities that do not incur expense nor are there any whose expense cannot be controlled to some extent. If cost were of no consideration, the quality of laboratory services could be carried to whatever level unlimited expenditures would provide. However, because of the customary financial constraints, efforts must be made continually to strike and hold the most effective balance between the quality and cost of services.

Cost control is the means by which this balance is maintained. Quality at any price is untenable and must be substituted by the more realistic practice of cost effectiveness. The following discussion includes those activities we feel are most pertinent to this area of laboratory responsibility.

To reliably plan and forecast laboratory expenditures, accurate projections of workload must first be made. These forecasts are preferably made on the number of tests rather than on revenues, which can be seriously misleading because of price changes.

The growth rate (percent) of each laboratory procedure is determined for the preceding year and, by applying this

GENERAL PRINCIPLES

FORECAST OF WORKLOAD

rate to the preceding year's volume, one can project the number of tests for each new fiscal year. Forecasts of new tests to be introduced and those whose volume may be affected by changes in laboratory strategy are also made. Because physician utilization is less predictable, these projections will be less reliable. (See Appendix B for Projected Workload form.)

FORECAST OF EXPENDITURES

The forecast of expenditures necessary to perform the anticipated workload over a designated time period is termed a budget. It is a strong management tool by which organizational objectives may be achieved through planned and controlled expenditures.

The budget may be perceived as the foundation of all cost control programs since it exercises broad constraints on total organizational expenditures. Effective budgeting requires careful identification of all categories of expenditures and the most prudent allocation of funds for each. A meaningful budget must be accurate and closely adhered to. Budgets most commonly encompass one year, but expenditure projections beyond this twelve-month period are highly desirable.

The grouping of expense categories for budgetary purposes is often termed a "chart of accounts." A proposed hospital laboratory chart of accounts follows:

1. Salaries
   A. Exempt
   B. Nonexempt
2. Supplies
3. Equipment
   A. Purchase
   B. Rental
   C. Lease
   D. Maintenance
   E. Depreciation
4. Reference laboratory fees
5. Continuing education and travel
6. Subscriptions and dues
7. Hospital administrative assistance
8. Telephone
9. Housekeeping

10. General mainte-
    nance
11. Electricity
12. Building deprecia-
    tion
13. Taxes
    A. Payroll
    B. Sales
14. Insurance
    A. General liability
    B. Workman's
       Compensation
    C. Group health
    D. Other
15. Miscellaneous

Laboratory budgeting is an ongoing process that culmi-
nates annually with the expense projections for the forthcoming fiscal year. The forecasts are made in accordance
with the chart of accounts and are divided into quarters.
We feel these three-month intervals represent the best
times for expenditure modifications. (See the Budget Form
in Appendix B.)

WORKLOAD AND REVENUE REPORTS

During the course of each fiscal year, quarterly workload
and revenue reports are submitted to the department.
These are generally provided by the hospital administration and include both the projected and actual figures for
each laboratory within the department and their deviations
for the most recent quarter and the year to date. (See
Appendix B for Workload and Revenue Report form.)

BUDGET REPORTS

As with workload and revenue reports, the department is
provided with quarterly budget reports. These include the
actual and projected expense figures for each laboratory in
the department with their deviations for the most recent
quarter and the year to date. In addition to the broad
controls implicit in the budgeting process, these quarterly
reports provide a means for periodically monitoring actual
expenditures and determining the reasons for any deviations that occur. (See Appendix B for the Budget Report
form.)

119

CAPITAL EQUIPMENT EXPENDITURES

In accordance with the policy of most hospitals, capital equipment is any instrument that costs more than $100.00. Because of potentially large expenditures and the number of options and alternatives afforded, a studied approach to the selection and method of acquisition of such equipment is dictated.

Planning for these expenditures may be divided into two stages. The first is developing an awareness of new equipment having potential application within the laboratory. This stage may be considered a time of general investigation, which is greatly facilitated by maintaining a file of new product information.

The second stage is consideration of annual recommendations for new equipment acquisition. These recommendations must be accompanied by descriptions, prices, sources, justification, and priority of need. (See Appendix B for a Capital Equipment Request form.)

Capital expenditure is an investment. As such its rate of return must be evaluated and used as a criterion for budgeting decisions (see Chapter 12 on the cost of capital and capital budgeting). Suggested categories of justification and priority of need are as follows:

Justification categories
  A. Replacement—equipment cannot be repaired, or excessive cost of repair results in unacceptable delays in service
  B. Increased workload—volume increase justifies either automation or additional personnel
  C. Cost reduction—reduction of operational expenses stated primarily in terms of personnel and supplies
  D. New and/or improved methodology—better patient care

Priority of need
  A. Essential—needed immediately to maintain quality patient care

B. Necessary—as "essential," but greater leeway with regard to time of acquisition
C. Desirable—means of reducing costs
D. Other—means of improving general working conditions

SALARIES

Personnel costs invariably constitute the largest expenditure of the hospital laboratory. Because of this expense, efforts to constantly assure the most efficient employment and deployment of the staff are of major importance in controlling laboratory costs. These efforts are concerned basically with the selection, distribution, and utilization of these persons. For a closer analysis of the methods for achieving these objectives, see Chapter 3, Organizing and Staffing the Hospital Laboratory.

PURCHASE AND UTILIZATION OF SUPPLIES

Efficient procurement of supplies is essential to every meaningful and effective hospital laboratory cost control program. All needs must be accurately identified and clearly communicated in sufficient time to avoid or minimize shortages and expensive interruptions in services.

The procurement of laboratory supplies is greatly facilitated by an inventory system that identifies all supply needs and the quantity of these items to be kept immediately available. In addition, the system must allow personnel both a means of identifying depletions and the means for triggering timely replacements. It must be closely monitored, periodically updated, and kept sufficiently flexible to easily admit, delete, or modify the quality and quantity of all items so dicated by changing methodology and usage.

The heart of such a system is the inventory card. Each item is assigned one such card on which there are spaces for recording the quantities on hand. Minimum and maximum numbers are also listed on the card along with the quantity to be stocked. Whenever depletions result in a balance equaling the minimum number, an order is promptly initiated to replenish the item to its maximum number. (See Appendix B for recommended inventory card format.)

Carefully monitored supply costs constitute a major opportunity to control hospital laboratory expenses. Although a variety of methods may be employed, we recommend a system that relates supply costs to the total revenues.

The relationship of the costs and revenues may be computed as a ratio or percentage and stated for the entire department, each laboratory, or individual tests. The decision as to what percentage or ratio of total charges should be constituted by supply costs must be somewhat arbitrary and individualized for each laboratory. Once a prudent decision is reached, however, every effort must be made not to exceed the established figure. Whenever such efforts fail, the responsible tests must be reviewed and modified, replaced, or their price revised upward, in that order.

Given the alternatives mentioned above, we recommend monitoring supply costs by laboratory rather than by total department or individual tests. There are two reasons for this recommendation: (1) The necessary figures are easily obtained quarterly from the revenue and budget reports mentioned earlier in this chapter. (2) Financial reports by laboratory are sufficiently contracted and manageable to permit rapid pursuit and correction of the problem. If the same ratio analysis is applied to the entire department neither deviations nor specific problems are as promptly identified; the same analysis applied to individual tests is excessively detailed and no more informative.

PART FOUR

Modern financial concepts

11

FINANCIAL PLANNING

Financial planning involves a thorough understanding of the status quo, a look into the future, and an attempt to control those aspects that are controllable. It requires the wisdom to imagine the unfolding of long-term events, the courage to design and control, and, most difficult of all, the willingness to sacrifice short-lived gains for more lasting benefits.

In today's dynamic business environment, financial planning is vital to the survival of laboratories. As the economy grows more diverse with the emergence of new technology, there is such a multiplicity of possibilities that it is impossible not to plan. The bigger and the more successful the laboratories are, the more complex and demanding the planning processes are likely to become.

The hospital laboratory should be thought of as a profit center or business unit of the hospital. In the following section a sample planning model will be suggested and illustrated for the expansion of the production capacity through the conversion of Technicon's SMA to SMAC.

FINANCIAL PLANNING FOR THE HOSPITAL LABORATORY

The hospital laboratory is a unique and complex business. Often it is thought of as a service-rendering unit of the hospital. As a business, it is also like a manufacturing enterprise. Unfortunately, it has the least advantageous characteristics of both a manufacturing industry and a service firm. Its special features are:

1. *Service industry with heavy assets.* It has to produce—manufacture, as it were—clinical information. The production of laboratory data requires a heavy investment in assets such as scientific instruments and advanced technological facilities. Such heavy endowment of assets is more characteristic of a manufacturing concern than of a service firm.

2. *Extremely short service turn-around time.* It has to service physicians and patients within a short span of time. The constraint in time requires constant and demanding management of human and financial resources.

3. *Constant technological innovation.* It is in the forefront of technological innovation. The frequent changes and improvements in the techniques and methods of producing laboratory results create much uncertainty in the acquisition of equipment and material, which generally have a fast rate of obsolescence.

4. *Highly seasonal.* It is a seasonal business. Seasonality should be an important planning factor, especially in efforts to deploy the usually limited human and financial resources.

The operation of a hospital laboratory is akin to that of a bakery. Its complex features are cast against the flux of the economy to produce a tremendous number of uncertainties and possibilities. In the 1970s the dramatic rise in inflation to as high as 12% per year not only made capital more expensive to acquire, but also caused the rapid rise in prices for all sectors of the economy and the fall of profit margin in the medical laboratory industry. Such an environment calls for imaginative financial planning processes if resources for achieving the service goals are to be prudently deployed.

A viable financial planning model should evolve around the following three parts:
1. The evolution of a set of goals and objectives from an idea
2. The selection and design of policies and programs to achieve the objectives and goals
3. The implementation of the policies and programs (including a feedback mechanism) to monitor progress; the changing of plans to cope with unexpected events when necessary

The first two steps are strategic in nature, hence strategic planning. The third step is commonly known as operations.

Idea generation

The first step in financial planning is the generation of an idea (Fig. 11-1). This is by far the most difficult step. The simpler the idea is, the more elusive to imagination it becomes. The idea chosen must not only be potentially feasible economically, but it must also be of sufficient priority. For our model illustration, we will assume that a hospital laboratory is considering replacing its SMA with SMAC (Fig. 11-2). Idea generation for the laboratory is normally the duty of the laboratory director.

Goal definition

The chosen idea is not meaningful unless a goal or a set of goals is designed. The goal must be defined in terms of measurable tasks. For our idea of replacing SMA with SMAC, Fig. 11-3 shows the set of goals: (1) to decrease the cost per test of the sequential multiple analysis and (2) to increase the operational capacity. It must be understood that goals 1 and 2 are mutually exclusive, which says that meeting goal 1 does not necessarily mean the successful completion of the other. If mutual exclusivity is not the case, we are really defining a single goal in two different ways.

127

FIG. 11-1
Ideas for the hospital laboratory.

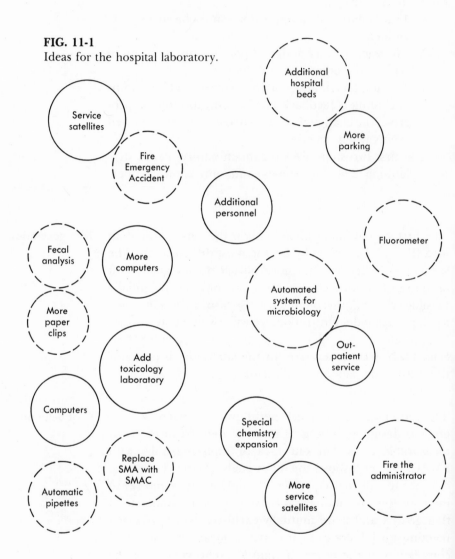

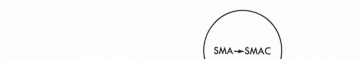

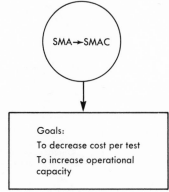

FIG. 11-2
The birth of an idea.

FIG. 11-3
Goal definition.

Objective definition

The next step is the definition of objectives. These are components or "subgoals," so to speak. Each objective is designed to be independently evaluated. When all the objectives are fully conceived, we will have set the stage to realize the goal(s). The objectives must be defined with measurable characteristics. In our illustration, we have defined the following three objectives with their measurable implications (Fig. 11-4): (1) Current SMA efficiency, (2) financial, market, and operational changes, and (3) future SMAC efficiency. In addition to the measurable characteristics, the set of objectives must also fulfill the qualifying condition of completeness. In our model illustration, it will require a positive answer to the question: Will the set of objectives together yield sufficient information for the hospital laboratory director to decide whether to replace the SMA with the SMAC? If the answer is negative, then the set of objectives is incomplete.

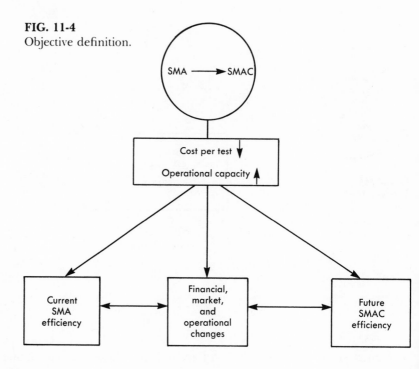

FIG. 11-4
Objective definition.

The analysis cycle   This cycle consists of two steps, which may be iterative (Fig. 11-5). For the fulfillment of the objective of current SMA efficiency, we formulate a set of desired SMA efficiency parameters. We then collect sufficient data to derive these parameters. The characteristics of these parameters are: (1) they are factual; (2) they are most meaningful when we examine them collectively; individually they may not appear relevant; and (3) they are related to each other. The data analyses should show such a relationship. If they do not, then some or all of the data gathered may not be sensitive to the chosen efficiency parameters. Such a negative condition requires another iteration of the analysis cycle. For our SMA efficiency parameters, the following may, for example, be formulated:

FIG. 11-5
The analysis cycle.

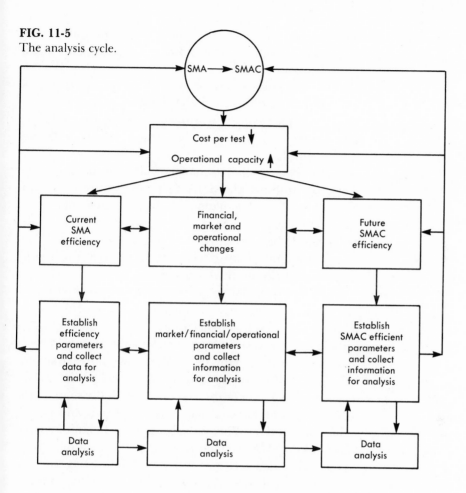

1. The monthly volume of specimens in the last three months
2. The manhours per week in the last thirteen weeks spent in running the SMA unit
3. The ratios of down-time to up-time and idle-time to up-time in the last three months

It is worth noting that the link among the three efficiency parameters is the specified time, i.e., three months.

The parameters may not show any significant trend because the length of time chosen may be too short or the SMA operation may have already passed the growth phase (see the next section on Growth Pattern). Therefore, we may wish to lengthen the time frame and repeat the analysis cycle. It may even be worthwhile to compare the longer time frame with a similar time frame in the preceding twelve months.

A subsequent analysis may show that the manhours per week for running the SMA unit are relatively constant regardless of the fluctuations of the specimen volume. In this event, the manhour criterion as an efficiency parameter is said to be insensitive. An insensitive parameter is either redundant or insufficient in depth. If it can not be improved, it should be discarded.

The future SMAC efficiency may be evaluated with a similar set of efficiency parameters as those of the SMA. However, market, financial, and operational changes should have measurable parameters that would answer questions such as: How large is the current market for automated chemistry specimens? What will be the growth rate of this segment of the market? What is the share of the market for the hospital laboratory? What would be the initial cash outlay? What is the break-even point for changing SMA to SMAC? What is the expected cost of capital? What is the quarterly or yearly cash inflow? Is the current price justifiable? What would be the impact of a cost reduction? Some of these questions are dealt with in Chapters 12 and 13.

Decision junctures

The last step in financial planning is to assemble sufficient information for decision-making (Fig. 11-6). The information should answer the question: Is the idea feasible from the market, financial, and operational points of view? In our example, it should demonstrate whether or not, by

FIG. 11-6
Decision junctures.

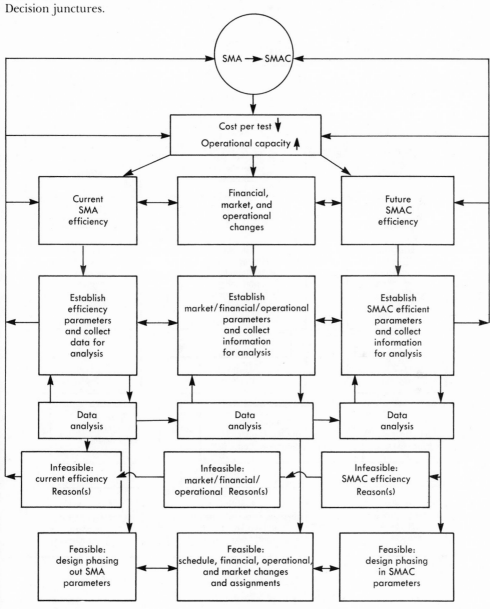

FIG. 11-7
The idea in action.

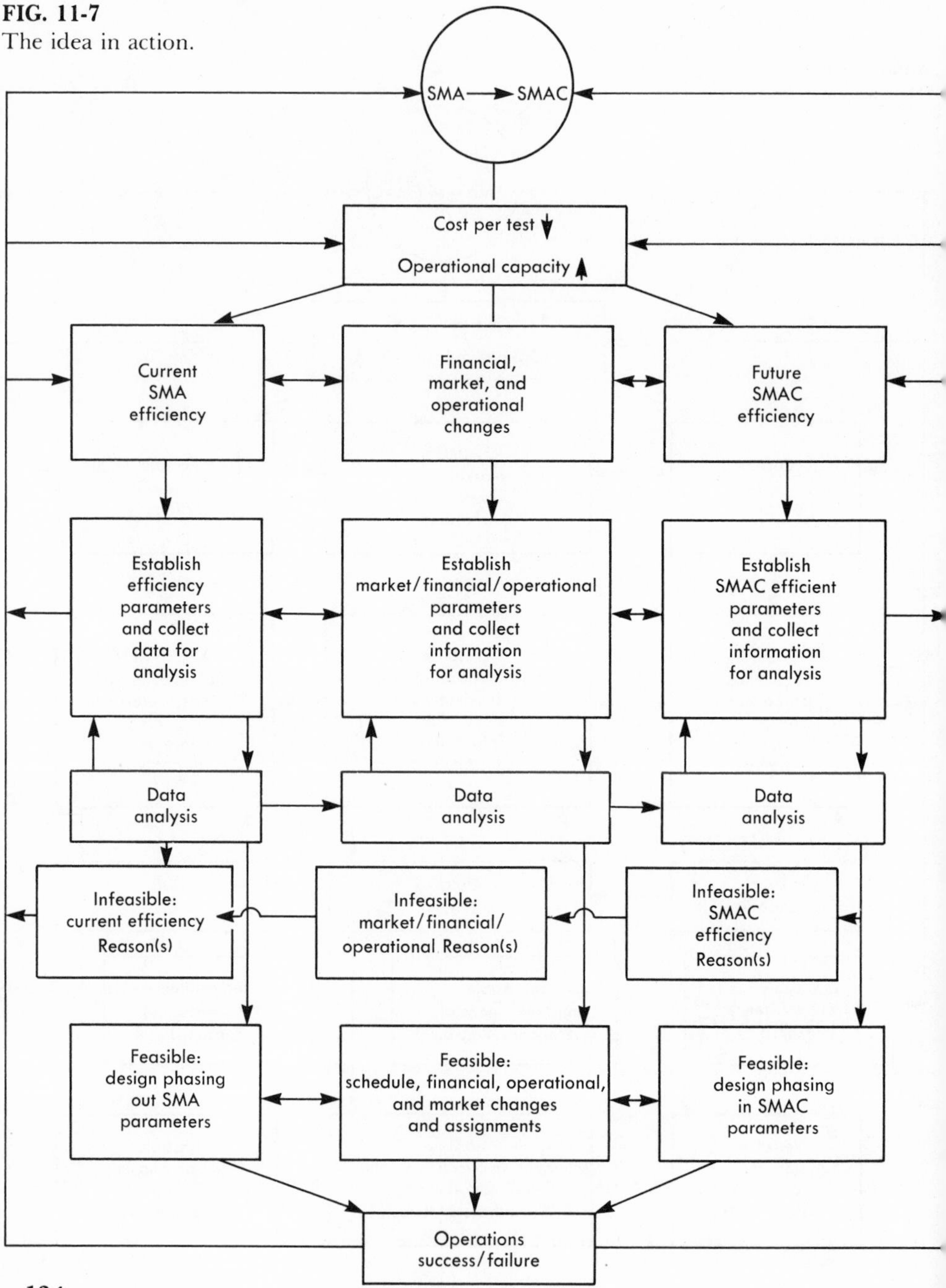

switching SMA to SMAC, there will be a consequential reduction in cost per test and/or an increase in operational capacity. By answering the questions of the preceding section we will have the information we need for the feasibility study step. When we know the cash inflow, the cost of capital, and cash outflow, the idea should then be subjected to a present value or an internal rate of return analysis (see Chapter 12).

The entire planning model from the conception of an idea to operations is summarized in Fig. 11-7. The model is intended to stimulate the reader's thinking concerning planning processes pertinent to the management of hospital laboratories.

We shall conclude this chapter with a discussion of the concepts of growth patterns and break-even analysis, which will shed some light on the service industry characteristics of the hospital laboratory.

GROWTH PATTERN

The growth of a laboratory, a product, or a technology usually follows the configuration shown in Fig. 11-8. Such a growth pattern can be considered as having four phases. Phase I depicts the start-up stage, which usually is not yet profitable. The rate of growth, corresponding to the slope

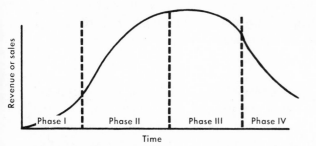

FIG. 11-8
The product life cycle or growth pattern.

of the Phase I portion of the curve, is also sluggish and may even be discouraging to those who have never experienced any start-up venture. This is also the phase in which more laboratory or product failures occur. Financial planning for this phase is most difficult and challenging because of the many inherent uncertainties.

Phase II is the growth phase. This phase has the greatest operational agony. As indicated by the accelerated rate of growth, this is the phase of fastest expansion. It is also during this phase that a laboratory venture breaks even or a product begins to pay off. The chance of its long-term survival is considered much improved if it has successfully weathered this phase of the operation. Financial planning during this phase is most exciting because of the unusual growth rate even though there is still much uncertainty.

Phase III is the mature stage. Operational pains are usually no longer as great as those of Phase II. The growth rate also has slowed from the previous stage. When a laboratory has achieved this phase of growth, its chance of survival is considered most favorable. Financial planning for Phase III becomes a routine and continuous necessity.

The fourth phase of growth is really negative growth. It is the decline of the laboratory, technology, or product. This portion of the growth pattern should present a challenge to the hospital laboratory. At the very least, it should be anticipated so that it will trigger a search for a new product or technology.

**BREAK-EVEN
ANALYSIS**

Break-even analysis is the study of the relationship among the fixed cost, the variable cost, and profit. The units of production are compared with the total revenue. The link between the units of production and the total revenue is, of course, the price. However, if there are many products or kinds of services, the link then becomes the weighted average price of the products or services (see Appendix C, weighted average).

Fig. 11-9 depicts a typical break-even analysis. Assuming that the total cost (C) is a linear function of the fixed cost (F) and the variable cost (V), then

$$C = F + V \qquad \text{(11-1)}$$

Let us also assume that the total revenue (R) is a linear function of the price (P) and the units sold *(x)*. Then

$$R = xP \qquad \text{(11-2)}$$

At break-even point, we have

$$C = R \qquad \text{(11-3)}$$

or

$$xP = F + V \qquad \text{(11-4)}$$

which yields

$$x = \frac{F + V}{P} \qquad \text{(11-5a)}$$

or

$$P = \frac{F + V}{x} \qquad \text{(11-5b)}$$

Equation 11-5a gives us an example of the number of units of production to be sold for breaking even when the price is known. The break-even price can be estimated

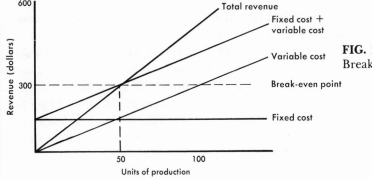

FIG. 11-9
Break-even analysis.

TABLE 11-1

Fixed cost and variable cost

Fixed cost	Variable cost
Depreciation on facility and equipment	Production labor
Rentals	Material
Interest charges	Sales commissions
Salaries	
General office expense (overhead)	

using equation 11-5b when one wishes x to be the units sold to break even. (See Chapter 13 for a more comprehensive approach to pricing.)

Table 11-1 describes the usual items under fixed cost and variable cost. A service industry typically has very few fixed assets compared with a manufacturing concern. Its fixed cost, therefore, becomes minimal, making the break-even point much lower than that of a manufacturing firm. Thus a service industry requires a much smaller total revenue than a manufacturing concern to break even. The two cases are briefly illustrated in Figs. 11-10 and 11-11.

It is traditional to think of the hospital laboratory as a service-rendering part of the hospital. From the financial point of view, the service-rendering features have been burdened by modern technological advances to include a heavy acquisition of fixed assets involving large capital outlay in the purchase of automated equipment, spectrophotometers, cell counters, tissue processors, etc. The necessary capital expenditures raise the fixed cost level, which in turn elevates the break-even point.

In addition, when we closely examine the items in Table 11-1 for the hospital laboratory, we find that the only item that resembles a variable cost is material or supplies. This usually amounts to 10 to 15 percent of the total budget for the laboratory, much of which may not even be controllable. The greater part of the total cost is more closely analo-

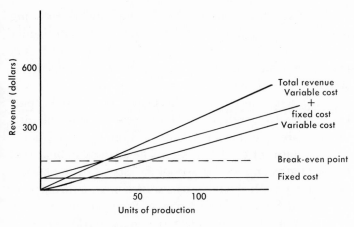

FIG. 11-10
Break-even analysis for a service firm.

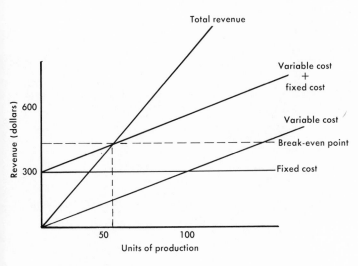

FIG. 11-11
Break-even analysis for a manufacturing firm.

gous to fixed cost. This has the effect of further elevating the break-even point of the laboratory operation. Under such a circumstance, there are few financial parameters in either the fixed cost or the variable cost that can yield to any system for financial control.

In practical terms, financial planning for the hospital laboratory involves the continuous gathering and analyzing of accurate and pertinent information to establish the current status of the laboratory. The analysis should yield the strengths and weaknesses of all aspects of the laboratory operation. It should also be sufficiently comprehensive to be used for predictive purpose. From the information gathered one should be able to obtain a better background for the financial decision-making process. Projections of future events, such as growth patterns, break-even analysis, profit planning, etc., are necessarily continuous financial functions.

12

COST OF CAPITAL AND CAPITAL BUDGETING

Before we can discuss capital budgeting we must consider the cost of capital. The word "capital" refers to the financial resources available for the firm or business unit. It can be generated internally as well as externally. The sources for internal capital are retained earnings and amounts paid in by the shareholders of the firm. External sources of funds are the capital market, such as banks and credit companies, and the public and private investors, such as insurance companies, individuals, and groups of investors. External sources of funds normally require a return of the principal plus interest. The interest charged for such external source of capital then becomes the *cost* of capital. Similarly, the shareholders of a business such as the hospital are entitled to some return on their investment. The rate of such a return is also a kind of cost of capital. For a nonprofit hospital or institution, the cost of capital is also pertinent in the sense that the assets should return a minimal amount in order to preserve their purchasing power.

Inflation is the erosion of the purchasing power of capital. In a no-growth situation, capital assets should earn a rate of return equal to at least the rate of inflation or the cost of capital, whichever is higher. During the 1970s the cost of capital has been inflating, thus requiring a greater rate of return for investment projects. As inflation rates soared to as high as 12 percent in recent years compared to 1.5 to 2 percent in the 1950s and early 1960s, the lending rates were driven up causing a tremendous increase in the cost of capital.

The interest structure of the capital market serves as an adequate measure for the cost of capital, which, in turn, allows the sophisticated businessman to base the rate of return. A given market interest rate reflects minimally the risk-free rate, which is the rate of interest on U.S. Government securities. Additionally, it may include the business risk and the financial risk. For a successful business, the rate of return should not only reflect the cost of capital but also additional rate of return for growth.

COMPOUND INTEREST

The concept of compound interest is, or should be, fundamental to sophisticated business thinking. Yet it is not unusual to find the very concept eluding successful business executives. This trend of "success in spite of oneself," however, may be fading as more and more firms desire to maintain a reasonable degree of growth and as the price for growth (the cost of capital) remains at a historically high level.

The subject of compound interest is not as difficult to understand as it may seem. In its simplest form, it can be expressed as

$$P_n = P_0 (1 + i)^n \tag{12-1}$$

where

P_n = the sum value of the principle and interest at the end of the nth period

P_0 = the value or principle at the beginning or the initial amount at time 0

i = the interest rate for each period

n = the number of periods, years, months, etc. (sometimes known as the time horizon)

chapter 12

Cost of capital and capital budgeting

Example 1. If we have $1.00 deposited in a savings account which yields an annual interest of 5 percent and is compounded annually, what is the amount at the end of four years?

At the end of four years

P_4 = $1.00 × (1 + 0.05)^4
    = $1.00 × 1.05 × 1.05 × 1.05 × 1.05
    = $1.216
    = $1.22 rounded off to the nearest cent

Table C-1 in Appendix C provides the interest factor or the value of $(1 + i)^n$ for $1.00 when i and n are known. When using the table, equation 12-1 becomes

$P_n = P_0 (F)$ **(12-2)**

where

    $F = (1 + i)^n$ = the interest factor

Example 2. If we deposit $2,000 in a credit union that pays 8 percent yearly interest compounded annually, what is the amount at the end of seven years?

$P_7 = \$2,000 × (1.08)^7$

Table C-1 gives us 1.714 as the interest factor of $1.00 at 8 percent for seven periods. Therefore

P_7 = $2,000 × 1.714
    = $3,428

Example 3. If the same credit union in example II decides to compound the interest quarterly, what will be the amount in seven years?

At the end of seven years, the account will have been compounded 28 times (4 × 7). However, the interest rate at the end of each period or quarter will be 2 percent (8 ÷ 4). This is equivalent to

$P_{28} = \$2,000 × (1 + 0.02)^{28}$

Table C-1 gives us the interest factor of 1.741 for 2 percent for 28 periods. Therefore

$$P_{28} = \$2,000 \times 1.741$$
$$= \$3,482$$

PRESENT VALUE The P_0 in equation 12-1 is also known as the present value and the P_n the future value. Rewriting equation 12-1 in terms of the present value, we have

$$P_0 = \frac{P_n}{(1 + i)^n}$$

which becomes

$$P_0 = P_n \left[\frac{1}{(1 + i)^n} \right] \tag{12-3}$$

We now have an expression that allows us to convert future streams of revenue to their present equivalent. This conversion is also known as discounting, which is simply the reverse of compounding. The discounting technique is very useful in comparing the worth of future receipts to the value of the current required investment.

Equation 12-3 can be rewritten as

$$P_0 = P_n D \tag{12-4}$$

where

$$D = \text{present value factor} = \frac{1}{(1 + i)^n}$$

The present value factors for \$1.00 in the future at different interest rates for n periods are tabulated in the Table C-2 of Appendix C.

Example 4. Suppose someone offers you either \$800 now or \$1,000 six years from now. You know that the future payment is certain. Furthermore, you also know that if you have the money now, you can deposit it in a savings account to earn 4 percent interest. Which amount should you accept?

$$P_0 = \$1,000 \; \frac{1}{(1 + 0.04)^6}$$
$$= \$1,000 \times 0.790$$
$$= \$790$$

Therefore, you should accept the $800 offer. We can alternatively arrive at the same conclusion by comparing the future value

$$\$800 \times (1 + 0.04)^6 = \$1,012$$

which is greater than $1,000 at the end of six years.

DETERMINING INTEREST RATES

If the present value and the future cash flow are known, the interest rate can be calculated by the following rearrangement of equation 12-2.

$$P_n = P_0 (1 + i)^n = P_0 F$$

$$\frac{P_n}{P_0} = F \qquad\qquad \textbf{(12-5a)}$$

Example 5. Suppose a bank agrees to lend you $1,000 if you sign a note promising to pay back $1,188 in two years. What is the rate of interest on the loan?

$$\frac{P_n}{P_0} = \frac{1,188}{1,000} = 1.188$$

From Table C-1 in Appendix C we can see that the interest rate closest to the interest rate factor of 1.188 in the compound value of $1.00 for two periods is 9%, which is the annual rate of interest charged by the bank.

Similarly, equation 12-4 can be rearranged to yield

$$\frac{P_0}{P_n} = D \qquad\qquad \textbf{(12-5b)}$$

**CAPITAL
BUDGETING** Budgeting really means that there is a scarcity of capital. There are two kinds of budgeting: operations and capital. Operations budgeting generally is a method used to allocate a limited amount of resources for maintaining the existing business. Capital budgeting, however, is a process of planning the spending of capital for projects that may yield benefits beyond one year. The one year criterion is more traditional than logical. However, it is a useful cut-off point for purposes of depreciation and accounting.

The concept of capital budgeting is often thought to be complex or conceptually difficult, but it need not be. However, there are four important factors that must be borne in mind when one makes any attempt at capital budgeting:

1. The result of the capital budgeting process is as accurate as the input information. If the input information is inferior, capital budgeting then becomes a wasted effort (i.e., the "garbage in—garbage out syndrome").
2. The supply of capital is usually limited and such limitation imposes upon a business enterprise a certain cost of capital.
3. The cash inflow in the future to the firm adequately serves as the basis for determining the allocation of capital.
4. There is uncertainty in the capital budgeting decision process because it is virtually impossible to know with absolute certainty the cost of capital or the stream of future cash inflow.

With these important factors in mind, we will discuss the common methods used in capital budgeting.

Payback method This traditional method requires that any investment be paid back as soon as possible or paid back within a specified period according to the hospital's policy. Table 12-1 shows the net cash flow of two investment projects.

146

Table 12-1

Net cash inflows for two investment projects

Year	Project A	Project B
1	$600	$100
2	400	200
3	200	400
4	100	800

Each requires an initial investment of $1,000. According to the payback method, Project A should be chosen because it will return the initial capital outlay in two years while Project B requires almost 3½ years.

The payback method is easy to calculate. However, it ignores the impact of the cash inflow beyond the payback period. It also conveniently by-passes the important notion of the firm's cost of capital. For long-term investments, the method can lead to the selection of less desirable projects. Surprisingly, it is still frequently the only method used by many major business firms.

Net present value (NPV) method

This method takes into consideration the business firm's cost of capital and the long-term effect of the cash inflow. The NPV model can be stated as follows:

$$NPV = \sum_{t=1}^{n} \frac{R_t}{(1 + k)^t} - C \qquad (12\text{-}6)$$

where

C = initial capital outlay
R_t = cash inflow in period t
k = cost of capital
t = time horizon = 1, 2, 3 .... n
n = the project's expected life

(If necessary, refer to the Appendix for the explanation of the sigma [Σ] symbol.)

Example 6. Calculate the NVP for Project A and Project B in Table 12-1 if the cost of capital is 10 percent. Assume that both projects have equal degrees of uncertainty. Which is a better investment?

Project A

$$NPV = \frac{600}{1.10} + \frac{400}{(1.10)^2} + \frac{200}{(1.10)^3} + \frac{100}{(1.10)^4} - 1,000$$
$$= 545 + 331 + 150 + 68 - 1,000$$
$$= \$94$$

Project B

$$NPV = \frac{100}{1.10} + \frac{200}{(1.10)^2} + \frac{400}{(1.10)^3} + \frac{800}{(1.10)^4} - 1,000$$
$$= 91 + 165 + 301 + 546 - 1,000$$
$$= \$103$$

Project B is a better investment.

In the present value approach, the minimal criterion for accepting an investment project is that its net present value be at least greater than zero. At $NPV = 0$, the future cash inflow will be just sufficient to cover the required cost of capital. Therefore, both Project A and Project B are acceptable at a 10% cost of capital. However, if these projects do not perform overlapping functions and if the business firm has insufficient capital to invest in both projects, then Project B is preferred.

Internal rate of return (IRR) method

It is sometimes convenient to rank investment projects according to their rates of return when we know their initial capital outlay and the corresponding future revenues. Under such a circumstance, equation 12-6 assumes the special case of zero net present value:

$$NPV = 0 = \sum_{t=1}^{n} \frac{R_t}{(1 + r)^t} - C \tag{12-7}$$

where r represents the internal rate of return. For a project to be acceptable as an investment, the internal rate of return r must be greater than the cost of capital k.

In evaluating investment projects, however, it is somewhat easier to compute the net present value using the cost of capital than to determine the internal rate of return. Also, the net present value method is preferred when ranking one investment project whose cost is much larger than that of another and when the timing of the projects' cash flows differs widely.

The tedium in capital budgeting is in the assembling of data for the estimation of cash outlay and of future revenues. In estimating the net initial capital outlay, we need to consider the purchase price of the new asset from which we should subtract the tax savings for the investment, if any, and the salvage value of the old machine or asset. Future revenues are determined by the sum of the additional profits and of depreciation benefits resulting from the anticipated new investment.

13

PRICING

The matter of pricing should be considered one of the few controllable options for the decision-making process of the laboratory management. It should be thoroughly exercised. Its planning should relate to the profit and loss of the laboratory as a cost center. Because of the importance of pricing to the long-term survival of the laboratory and the hospital, this entire chapter is devoted to the elaboration of a pricing model that should prove useful for evaluating new as well as existing procedures.

How does one price a laboratory procedure? Traditionally it has been done by guessing, second-guessing, or matching with another laboratory's prices. When the market place becomes competitive, random pricing not only complicates the guessing game, but adds confusion to planning efforts. The need for a logical pricing system is even more evident when one imagines the possibilities of third parties, government agencies, or consumer groups rightfully demanding some explanation for widely differing prices for a given procedure.

THE HEMMAPLARDH-SHUFFSTALL PRICING MODEL

The pricing model (HSPM) is essentially one of evaluating the inflow and outflow of cash and discounting the future flows by appropriate rates of return. We will illustrate our model one step at a time as we go through the example. It is our intention that the HSPM stimulate the systematic approach to laboratory pricing.

The HSPM in its simplest and most elegant form is expressed by the following:

$$\sum_{i=1}^{i=t} \frac{(NCF)_i}{(1 + r)^{i-1}} = 0$$

where

i = the time horizon in years ending in t^{th} year
r = the appropriate rate of return
NCF = cash inflow − cash outflow = net cash flow

CASH INFLOW

Let us consider the example of a hospital laboratory evaluating the proper price for serum protein electrophoresis. The first thing we need to know is the time horizon. Assume that the appropriate laboratory personnel have studied the situation and determined that the equipment such as the power supply unit, trays, etc., could be used for as long as five years, that is, $i = 1, 2, 3, 4, 5$. The summation (see Appendix C) will be performed on five terms. There will also be five sets of cash inflow and outflow.

The laboratory personnel have further estimated that the laboratory could conservatively expect 200, 400, 700, 900, and 1000 specimens, respectively, for each of the five consecutive years. Let x represent the initial dollar price of each serum protein electrophoresis specimen. The revenue for each year will be:

Initial cash flow estimates

Year 1	200x	Year 4	900x
Year 2	400x	Year 5	1000x
Year 3	700x		

Because inflation is expected, the hospital administration plans a 5 percent price increase each year. The revenues for the five years then become:

Cash inflow adjusted for price increase

Year 1	$200x$	$=$	$200x$
Year 2	$400x \times (1.00 + 0.005)$	$=$	$420x$
Year 3	$700x \times (1.00 + 0.05)^2$	$=$	$772x$
Year 4	$900x \times (1.00 + 0.05)^3$	$=$	$1,042x$
Year 5	$1,000x \times (1.00 + 0.05)^4$	$=$	$1,216x$

From the evaluation by the laboratory personnel, we know that the equipment will cost $4,000 and after five years the salvage value will be $500. We shall assume that the hospital is a corporation, subject to a 40% tax rate. The tax benefits from straight line depreciation (see Appendix C) will increase the cash flow for each of the five years to the following:

Cash inflow adjusted for price increase and depreciation

Year 1	$200x + (700 \times 0.4)$	$=$	$200x + 280$
Year 2	$420x + (700 \times 0.4)$	$=$	$420x + 280$
Year 3	$772x + (700 \times 0.4)$	$=$	$772x + 280$
Year 4	$1,042x + (700 \times 0.4)$	$=$	$1,042x + 280$
Year 5	$1,216x + (700 \times 0.4) + 500$	$=$	$1,216x + 780$

CASH OUTFLOW The laboratory further expects to allot ten hours each week of an employee's time to perform the electrophoresis, which presumably translates into $2,400 per year of direct labor cost. We will assume that the average laboratory worker's pay has been increasing at the rate of 6% per year. The cash outflow resulting from direct labor cost is:

Cash outflow attributed to labor

Year 1	$2{,}400 \times (1.00 + 0.00)$	$= 2{,}400$
Year 2	$2{,}400 \times (1.00 + 0.06)$	$= 2{,}544$
Year 3	$2{,}400 \times (1.00 + 0.06)^2$	$= 2{,}697$
Year 4	$2{,}400 \times (1.00 + 0.06)^3$	$= 2{,}858$
Year 5	$2{,}400 \times (1.00 + 0.06)^4$	$= 3{,}030$

Let us further assume that the hospital's chief financial officer has estimated that the overhead amounts to 50% of the direct labor cost. The cash outflow then becomes:

Cash outflow attributed to labor and overhead

Year 1	$2{,}400 \times 1.50$	$= 3{,}600$
Year 2	$2{,}544 \times 1.50$	$= 3{,}816$
Year 3	$2{,}697 \times 1.50$	$= 4{,}046$
Year 4	$2{,}858 \times 1.50$	$= 4{,}287$
Year 5	$3{,}030 \times 1.50$	$= 4{,}545$

At the initial phase of operation, there is a training or nonproductive period for which $400 will have to be expended. The cost of supplies is estimated to be $100, $130, $160, $180, and $200 for each of the successive five years. When the initial purchase price of $4,000 is included also in the cash outflow, we have:

Cash outflow attributed to labor, overhead, and others

Year 1	$3{,}600 + 400 + 4{,}000 + 100 = 8{,}100$
Year 2	$3{,}816 + 130 = 3{,}946$
Year 3	$4{,}046 + 160 = 4{,}206$
Year 4	$4{,}287 + 180 = 4{,}467$
Year 5	$4{,}545 + 200 = 4{,}745$

NET CASH FLOW   The net cash flow is the sum of the cash inflow minus the sum of the cash outflow. Therefore:

Net cash flow

Year 1	$(200x + 280) - 8,100 =$	$200x - 7,820$
Year 2	$(420x + 280) - 3,946 =$	$420x - 3,666$
Year 3	$(772x + 280) - 4,206 =$	$772x - 3,926$
Year 4	$(1,042x + 280) - 4,467 =$	$1,042x - 4,187$
Year 5	$(1,126x + 720) - 4,745 =$	$1,216x - 3,965$

THE RATE OF RETURN

The rate of return is the percentage of gain for a given investment. A profitable business must have the rate of return greater than the cost of capital. The management of a well-run hospital not only should have a firm grasp of its rate of return, but also should constantly monitor the fluctuations of the state of the economy in general and of its financial structure in particular, which would eventually have an impact on the rate.

The HSPM will be illustrated with different rates of return. However, for our first example, let us assume that the rate of return required of the serum protein electrophoresis investment is 12% per year.

PRICE AND PRICING IMPLICATIONS

The final form of our example of the model incorporating the 12 percent annual rate of return yields the following expression:

$$(200x - 7820) + \frac{420x - 3,666}{(1.00 + 0.12)} + \frac{772x - 3,926}{(1.00 + 0.12)^2}$$
$$+ \frac{1,042x - 4187}{(1.00 + 0.12)^3} + \frac{1216 - 3,965}{(1.00 + 0.12)^4} = 1216x$$

Solving for x, we obtain

$x = \$7.29.$

A good way to solve for x is the use of tabulation. The knowns and unknowns are separated into the right and left columns and discounting is applied to each as follows:

Tabulated pricing calculations

Year	Unknowns			Knowns		
1			$200x$			7,820
2	$420x$	$\div$ 1.12	$= 375x$	$3,666$	$\div$ 1.12	$= 3,273$
3	$772x$	$\div (1.12)^2$	$= 615x$	$3,926$	$\div (1.12)^2$	$= 3,130$
4	$1,042x$	$\div (1.12)^3$	$= 742x$	$4,187$	$\div (1.12)^3$	$= 2,980$
5	$1,216x$	$\div (1.12)^4$	$= 773x$	$3,065$	$\div (1.12)^4$	$= 2,520$
		Total	$2,705x$		Total	19,723

Therefore

$$2,705x = 19,723$$

$$\text{and } x = \frac{19,723}{2,705} = \$7.29$$

Alternatively, the calculations can be done by using the present value table (Table C-2). The price equation then becomes

$$(200x - 7,820) + (420x - 3,666)(0.893) +$$
$$(772x - 3,926)(0.797) + (1,042x - 4,187)(0.712) +$$
$$(1,216x - 3,965)(0.636) = 0$$

Multiplying and collecting terms, we have

$$2705x = 19,726$$
$$x = \$7.29$$

The price for a serum protein electrophoresis for each of the next five years is determined below:

Prices for serum protein electrophoresis

Year 1	\$7.29			
Year 2	\$7.29	$\times$ 1.05	$= \$7.65$	
Year 3	\$7.29	$\times (1.05)^2$	$= \$8.04$	
Year 4	\$7.29	$\times (1.05)^3$	$= \$8.44$	
Year 5	\$7.29	$\times (1.05)^4$	$= \$8.86$	

The impact of the varying rates of return on the first year price is similarly calculated (Table 13-1).

Table 13-2 illustrates the full implications of our model with six different rates of return. The yearly revenue is computed by using the initial volume estimates of 200, 400, 700, 900, and 1,000 specimens and the different yearly prices. Alternatively, the same annual revenue is obtained by multiplying the price for the first year of each rate of return with the adjusted specimen volumes or the coefficients of x as shown in the table on net cash flow.

Each line of the net outlay column is obtained by subtracting the yearly revenue from the yearly expense. Similarly, the net receipt line is obtained by subtracting the yearly expense from the yearly revenue.

At 0 percent rate of return, the pricing model gives us an idea of the floor price, so to speak. In this instance the accumulated outlay after two years is being returned with no appreciation at the end of five years. The slight difference between the accumulated outlay of $7,481 and the accumulated receipt of $7,496 resulted from the effects of rounding numbers in the calculations.

When the rate of return is greater than zero, the total outlay plus the annual return and adjusted for the time value of money is equal to the total receipt similarly

Table 13-1

First year price at different rates of return

Rate of return	First year price
0%	$ 6.46
12 %	$ 7.29
18 %	$ 7.74
24 %	$ 8.18
30 %	$ 8.65
76 %	$12.27

Serum protein electrophoresis pricing case summary

Rate of return (first year price)	Year	Yearly revenue	Accumulated revenue	Yearly expense	Accumulated yearly expense	Net outlay	Accumulated outlay	Net receipt	Accumulated receipt
0% ($6.46)	1st	$ 1,292	$ 1,292	$7,820	$ 7,820	$6,528	$6,528	None	None
	2nd	2,713	4,005	3,666	11,486	953	7,481	None	None
	3rd	4,987	8,992	3,926	15,412	None	None	$ 1,062	$ 1,062
	4th	6,731	15,723	4,187	19,599	None	None	2,544	3,606
	5th	7,855	23,578	3,965	23,564	None	None	3,890	7,496
12% ($7.29)	1st	$ 1,458	$ 1,458	$7,820	$ 7,820	$ 6,362	$ 6,362	None	None
	2nd	3,062	4,520	3,666	11,486	604	6,966	None	None
	3rd	5,628	10,148	3,926	15,412	None	None	$ 1,702	$ 1,702
	4th	7,596	17,744	4,187	19,599	None	None	3,409	5,111
	5th	8,865	26,609	3,965	23,564	None	None	4,900	10,011
18% ($7.74)	1st	$ 1,548	$ 1,548	$7,820	$ 7,820	$ 6,272	$6,272	None	None
	2nd	3,251	4,799	3,666	11,486	415	6,687	None	None
	3rd	5,975	10,774	3,926	15,412	None	None	$ 2,049	$ 2,049
	4th	8,065	18,839	4,187	19,599	None	None	3,878	5,925
	5th	9,412	28,251	3,965	23,564	None	None	5,447	11,372
24% ($8.18)	1st	$ 1,636	$ 1,636	$7,820	$ 7,820	$6,184	$6,184	None	None
	2nd	3,436	5,072	3,666	11,486	230	6,414	None	None
	3rd	6,315	11,387	3,926	15,412	None	None	$ 2,389	$ 2,389
	4th	8,524	19,911	4,187	19,599	None	None	4,337	6,726
	5th	9,947	29,858	3,965	23,564	None	None	5,982	12,708
30% ($8.65)	1st	$ 1,730	$ 1,730	$7,820	$ 7,820	$6,090	$6,090	None	None
	2nd	3,633	5,363	3,666	11,486	33	6,123	None	None
	3rd	6,678	12,041	3,926	15,412	None	None	$ 2,752	$ 2,752
	4th	9,013	21,054	4,187	19,599	None	None	4,826	7,578
	5th	10,518	31,572	3,965	23,564	None	None	6,553	14,131
76% ($12.27)	1st	$ 2,454	$ 2,454	$7,820	$ 7,820	$5,366	$5,366	None	None
	2nd	5,153	7,607	3,666	11,486	None	None	$ 1,487	$ 1,487
	3rd	9,472	17,079	3,926	15,412	None	None	5,546	7,033
	4th	12,785	29,864	4,187	19,599	None	None	8,598	15,631
	5th	14,920	44,784	3,965	23,564	None	None	10,955	26,586

adjusted. For example with 12 percent annual rate of return, the total adjusted outlay is

$$\$6,362 \times (1.12)^4 + \$604 \times (1.12)^3 = \$10,900$$

and the total adjusted receipt

$$\$1,702 \, (1.12)^2 + \$3,409 \times 1.12 + \$4.900 = \$10,900$$

The cash break-even point is the time at which the revenue equals expense. For the serum electrophoresis in our example such break-even points occur during the third year for 0, 12, 18, and 24 percent annual rates of return. However, the break-even points appear very early during the third year and sometime during the second year for rates of return of 30 and 76 percent, respectively, as indicated by the net outlay column. It is also worth noting that the accumulated outlay decreases as the rate of return increases.

The pricing model gives us another piece of extremely useful information in addition to price. From the net outlay column in Table 13-2 we can tell the amount of cash required for the investment in electrophoresis for each year at each price level. This information will allow both the hospital to plan for the required cash and the laboratory to better budget for its expenditure.

CONCLUDING REMARKS

Our pricing model is an example of a systematic approach to pricing. It is logically tenable. It also allows much flexibility because each step can be modified to a different situation in calculations for the cash inflow and outflow. The implied single rate of return will fluctuate because the rate of future inflation and the cost of money are expected to vary according to the state of the economy. However, our model should prove useful in many pricing situations, and it certainly represents an improvement over random pricing.

The expected changes in the rate of return can also be

treated as variations from the mean, the variance being a measure of uncertainty or risk. In such a circumstance, the rate of return must be increased to reflect the additional risk of the investment.

Each laboratory presumably is taxed at a different rate if it is not a nonprofit enterprise. Because of such uniqueness of each laboratory or hospital, the effect of taxation is purposely not explored in depth. This, however, can be easily incorporated into the streams of cash inflow and outflow for each year when the expected corporate tax rate is known with some certainty.

The HSPM approach can also be used for evaluating any existing procedure to determine whether it is appropriately priced, or alternately, whether it should be performed in-house. With the proper inputs, it can provide logical and justifiable trends for future prices, which are extremely useful in a competitive environment. Another equally important result of the pricing model is its generation of the required net cash outlay for each year at each price level, a piece of extremely useful management information that is normally difficult to obtain.

Appendixes

MANAGERIAL

Job title: Supervisor, Hematology Laboratory,
      Department of Laboratories
Date: January 1, 1978

I. Statement of the job
Under the supervision of the Technical and Administrative Coordinator, is responsible for the performance of all technical and administrative duties assigned to the Hematology Laboratory.

II. Duties of the job

1. Is responsible for the Hematology Laboratory being clean and orderly and work flow organized and efficient.

2. In consultation with the Technical and Administrative Coordinator and Directors, recommends and assists with selecting and developing all tests performed by the Hematology Laboratory; maintains up-to-date methodology manual that is constantly available for use and review by Hematology Laboratory personnel.

3. Supervises and assists with the performance of all procedures assigned to the Hematology Labora-

tory; is responsible for accuracy and clarity of reports.

4. In consultation with the Technical and Administrative Coordinator and Directors, is responsible for an efficient, effective, and documented quality control program within the Hematology Laboratory.

5. Sees that all job duties of Hematology Laboratory personnel are clearly defined and understood; is responsible for overall development, training, motivation, and performance of these same personnel.

6. Appraises and counsels all Hematology Laboratory personnel in order to improve total job performance; yearly, conducts formal job evaluation of all personnel in the Hematology Laboratory.

7. Interviews all applicants for job positions in the Hematology Laboratory; in consultation with the Technical and Administrative Coordinator and Directors, assists with hiring new personnel for the Hematology Laboratory; with same consultation, assists in all decisions concerning those personnel who fail to meet the standards of the Hematology Laboratory.

8. In consultation with the Technical and Administrative Coordinator, prepares and submits to the Director a budget of major expenses (number of personnel, supplies, and capital equipment) for each new fiscal year.

9. With Technical and Administrative Coordinator and Directors, reviews and analyzes all quarterly work volume and budget reports for the Hematology Laboratory.

10. In accordance with Department policy, is responsible for ordering all supplies for the Hematology Laboratory; constantly encourages efficient and

economical utilization of supplies by Hematology Laboratory personnel.

11. In consultation with the Technical and Administrative Coordinator, is responsible for an efficient, effective and documented preventive maintenance program for the Hematology Laboratory.

12. In consultation with the Technical and Administrative Coordinator, is responsible for the safety of all Hematology Laboratory personnel by assuring continuing compliance with the Department's safety program.

13. In consultation with the Educational Coordinator and Directors, is responsible for selecting and organizing all hematology lectures for the MLT school; is responsible for their presentation in accordance with lecture schedule.

14. Performs special assignments so indicated or approved by Director of Laboratories.

Job title: Technician, Hematology Laboratory,   **Technician**
          Department of Laboratories
Date: January 1, 1978

I. Statement of the job
   Under the direction of the Hematology Laboratory Supervisor, assists with all duties and responsibilities assigned to the Hematology Laboratory.

II. Duties of the job
   1. Assists in keeping work areas clean and orderly and work flow organized and efficient.
   2. Is proficient in the use of all equipment assigned to the Hematology Laboratory.
   3. Assists with the collection of laboratory specimens; in accordance with prescribed procedure, is pro-

ficient in the preparation of reagents, use of controls, and performance of all test methods assigned to the Hematology Laboratory.

4. Assists with the quality control and preventive maintenance programs of the Hematology Laboratory.
5. Is aware of and constantly complies with the Department's safety program.
6. Practices efficient and economical use of Hematology Laboratory supplies.
7. Assists with the hematology "bench" training of all MLT students.
8. Performs special assignments so indicated by the Hematology Laboratory Supervisor.

JOB SPECIFICATIONS

Supervisor

Job title: Supervisor, Hematology Laboratory, Department of Laboratories

Date: January 1, 1978

Factors	*Specifications*
1. Education	Must have minimum of two years of college; baccalaureate degree strongly preferred.
2. Certification	Must be certified as MT (ASCP).
3. Experience	Must have at least two years of experience in a Hematology Laboratory.
4. Orientation	Must learn details of job in 1-3 months; in 3-6 months, must be oriented to the attitudes and goals of the Department and effectively integrate the activities of the Hematology Laboratory into these total efforts.
5. Complexity of duties	Must understand the principles and be able to teach and perform all procedures assigned to the Hematology Laboratory; must be meticulous worker with an understanding of hematological

disorders; must be constantly alert to the quality and quantity of work performed in the Hematology Laboratory.

6. Independence of action

Must be able to carry out duties and responsibilities with minimal supervision.

7. Contact with others

Has close contact with Hematology Laboratory personnel and periodic contact with other supervisors, the Technical and Administrative Coordinator, Directors, physicians, and nursing personnel; must understand importance of effective communication and appreciate the necessity of coordinated efforts in attaining overall objectives.

8. Mental and visual demands

Requires a range of ability from understanding general concepts to skillfully performing test methods; must stay abreast of current hematology literature and evaluate and institute new methodology; must always seek methods for the improvement of services. Must perform moderate amount of microscopy.

9. Confidential data

Deals constantly with confidential medical information; must treat all such data with discretion.

10. Working conditions

Works in relatively crowded room with five other people and is subject to moderate traffic, noise, and interruptions; must be able to efficiently perform job duties under these circumstances.

11. Supervisory responsibility

Supervises five employees and instructs MLT students; must be aware of the daily demands placed on the Hematology Laboratory and the quality and rate of response by its personnel. Must exercise sound judgment and command respect; must effectively delegate some responsibility.

Technician

Job title: Technician, Hematology Laboratory,
Department of Laboratories
Date: January 1, 1978

Factors	*Specifications*
1. Education	Must have high school diploma; two years of college preferred.
2. Certification	Must be certified or eligible for certification by ASCP as MLT or CLA.
3. Experience	At least one year of experience in a Hematology Laboratory preferred; no experience would be considered.
4. Orientation	Must learn all job details in 3 months.
5. Complexity of duties	Must perform a variety of hematological procedures in strict accordance with the written methods of the Hematology Laboratory; must plan and organize work. Requires knowledge of and participation in the Department's quality control, preventive maintenance, and safety programs.
6. Independence of action	Performs under close supervision.
7. Contact with others	Works closely with supervisor and four other members of Hematology Laboratory; has limited contact with physicians and nursing personnel; must understand importance of effective communication and coordinated activities in attaining meaningful objectives.
8. Mental and visual demands	Requires close attention to many job duties and details. Uses microscope frequently; requires good vision and normal color perception.
9. Confidential data	Deals constantly with confidential medical information; must treat all such data with discretion.
10. Working conditions	Works in room with five other people and is subject to moderate noise, traffic, and interruptions. Must be able to efficiently perform job duties under these circumstances.
11. Supervisory responsibility	None. Assists with hematology "bench" training of MLT students.

OPERATING

A Cumulative Test Recording (CTR) system for laboratory quality control consists of 8×10 inch cards folded horizontally in half resulting in four sides, each 5×8 inches. The cards are placed in a Kardex file so that the patient identification information can be quickly recognized. Most such files permit up to forty-five cards per drawer (Fig. B-1).

Each of the four sides of the card includes a far lefthand column for the listing of tests and a series of additional columns to the right for dates and test results. Two patient identification information sites appear on side 1. The lower provides easy recognition while in the Kardex file. The upper is for quick retrieval when the card is alphabetically on end (Fig. B-2).

Results are recorded opposite the appropriate tests in successive left-to-right columns. At the time of each entry, the preceding results are immediately observed in the columns to the left. Folding a 8×10 inch card and using all four sides permits entry of a large number of tests and results, with a variety of arrangement options.

169

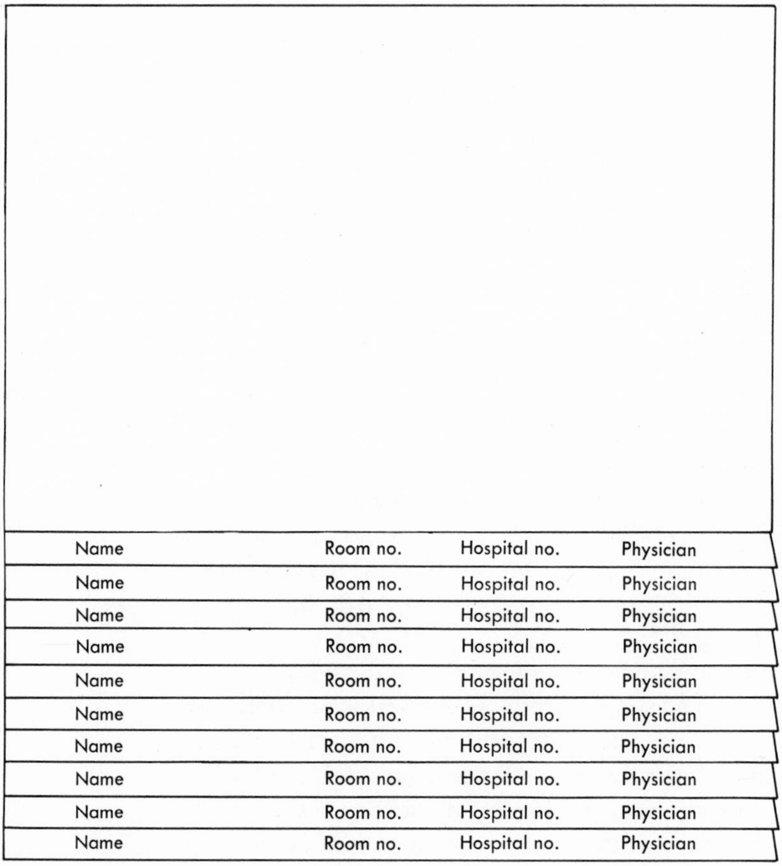

Name	Room no.	Hospital no.	Physician
Name	Room no.	Hospital no.	Physician
Name	Room no.	Hospital no.	Physician
Name	Room no.	Hospital no.	Physician
Name	Room no.	Hospital no.	Physician
Name	Room no.	Hospital no.	Physician
Name	Room no.	Hospital no.	Physician
Name	Room no.	Hospital no.	Physician
Name	Room no.	Hospital no.	Physician
Name	Room no.	Hospital no.	Physician

FIG. B-1

5 × 8 inch Kardex file with quickly discernible patient identification information.

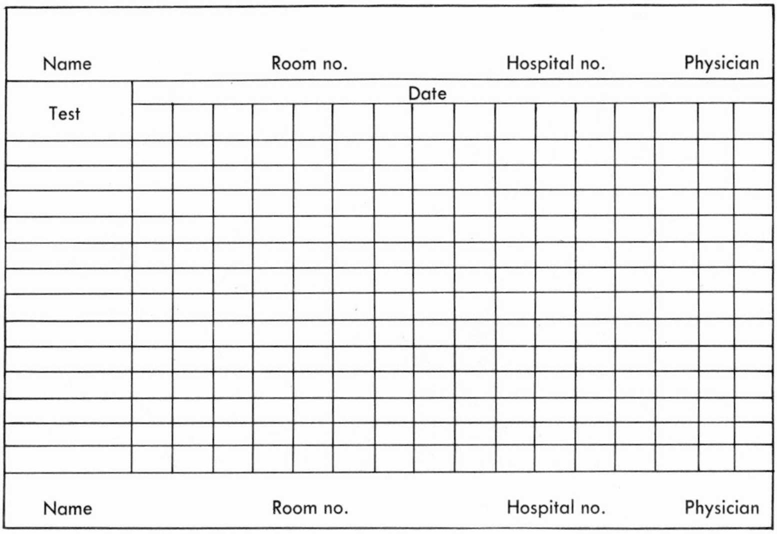

Name	Room no.	Hospital no.	Physician
Test	Date		

Name	Room no.	Hospital no.	Physician

FIG. B-2
Format of CTR card (side 1).

In the event the front surface of the 8 × 10 inch CTR card (sides 1 and 2) is insufficient to accommodate all test results, the back of the card is used (sides 3 and 4). This simply requires a reversal of the original rear fold to a forward fold, bottom to top. The side now foremost (side 3) includes patient information at its lower edge so that placement in the Kardex file continues to permit rapid identification (Fig. B-3).

The cards are entered into the Kardex file at the time of patient admission. Depending upon volume, they are easily alphabetized. At the time of discharge they are removed and filed alphabetically on end, side 1 foremost.

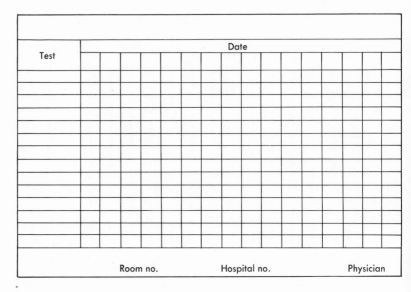

FIG. B-3
Format CTR card (side 2).

In addition to their contribution to quality control (by virtue of the analyst always being aware of preceding test results and avoiding reports of severely deviating results attributable to laboratory error), the CTR cards provide a convenient and compact copy of a patient's total laboratory record. As already noted, the card format permits modifications to suit all persuasions and circumstances.

Department of Laboratories
PERSONNEL EVALUATION FORM

Employee _____ Job title _____

Evaluation by _____ Job title _____

Period beginning _____ Period ending _____

Score by placing X in appropriate column.

Evaluation factors	<Ave.	Ave.*	>Ave.
Honesty—Displays a personal and professional integrity and conscientiousnes for always doing what is in the best interests of entire organization. Includes attendance and punctuality.			
Ambition—Displays willingness and desire to meet standards for quality and quantity of all job duties. Includes attire and personal appearance			
Initiative—Displays desire and ability to learn and achieve in excess of job duties so assigned.			
Determination—Displays desire and ability to perform all assigned job duties despite any difficulties encountered.			
Enthusiasm—Displays interest in and enjoyment from both the challenge and accomplishment of job duties.			
Common sense—Learns quickly from past laboratory experiences and applies these lessons in the best interests of the organization.			
Knowledge—Identifies factual and valid technical data and embodies a large amount of such data pertinent to his or her area of responsibility.			
Originality—Displays curiosity for what might be improved. Offers frequent valid suggestions for increasing the efficiency and effectiveness of assigned job duties.			
Understanding—Recognizes importance of teamwork to effectiveness of laboratory efforts. Maintains good relations with patients and all hospital and laboratory personnel.			
Communicative ability—Recognizes importance of good communication. Imparts all information clearly and concisely and listens attentively and observes carefully until all messages are understood.			

*Ave. (average) is level of performance of majority of employees as judged by employee and person conducting evaluation.

Employee _____ Evaluation by _____

       Signature   Signature

DAILY WORKSHEET—CHEMISTRY

Date _____

Patient	Rm.	Lab no.	Test no.	Instrument reading			Calculations	Results	Tech.
				Std.	Control	Test			

PREVENTIVE MAINTENANCE—DAILY

———— Laboratory

Month/Year

Equipment	Action no.	Action taken	1	2	3	4	5	6	7	8	9	10	11	12	13	14	15	16
Instrument A	1	[Statement of action]																
	2																	
	3																	
	4																	
	5																	
	6																	
	7																	
	8																	
	9																	
	10																	
Instrument B	1	[Statement of action]																
	2																	
	3																	
	4																	
Instrument C	1	[Statement of action]																
	2																	
Instrument D	1	[Statement of action]																
	2																	
	3																	
Instrument E	1	[Statement of action]																
	2																	
Instrument F	1	[Statement of action]																
	2																	
Instrument G	1	[Statement of action]																
	2																	
	3																	
Instrument H	1	[Statement of action]																
	2																	
	3																	

See weekly PM schedule

Continued.

PREVENTIVE MAINTENANCE—DAILY—cont'd

_____ Laboratory

Month/Year _____

Equipment	Action no.	Action taken	17	18	19	20	21	22	23	24	25	26	27	28	29	30	31
Instrument A	1	[Statement of action]															
	2																
	3																
	4																
	5																
	6																
	7																
	8																
	9																
	10																
Instrument B	1	[Statement of action]															
	2																
	3																
	4																
Instrument C	1	[Statement of action]															
	2																
Instrument D	1	[Statement of action]															
	2																
	3																
Instrument E	1	[Statement of action]															
	2																
Instrument F	1	[Statement of action]															
	2																
Instrument G	1	[Statement of action]															
	2																
	3																
Instrument H	1	[Statement of action]															
	2																
	3																

See weekly PM schedule

PREVENTIVE MAINTENANCE—WEEKLY

———— Laboratory

Year ————

Equipment	Action no.	Action taken	1	2	3	4	5	6	7	8	9	10	11	12	13
Instrument A	11	[Statement of action]													
	12														
Instrument B	5	[Statement of action]													
	6														
Instrument E	3	[Statement of action]													
	4														

See monthly PM schedule ————

See monthly and quarterly PM schedule ————

Equipment	Action no.	Action taken	14	15	16	17	18	19	20	21	22	23	24	25	26
Instrument A	11	[Statement of action]													
	12														
Instrument B	5	[Statement of action]													
	6														
Instrument E	3	[Statement of action]													
	4														

See monthly PM schedule ————

See monthly and quarterly PM schedule ————

See bi-yearly PM schedule ————

Continued.

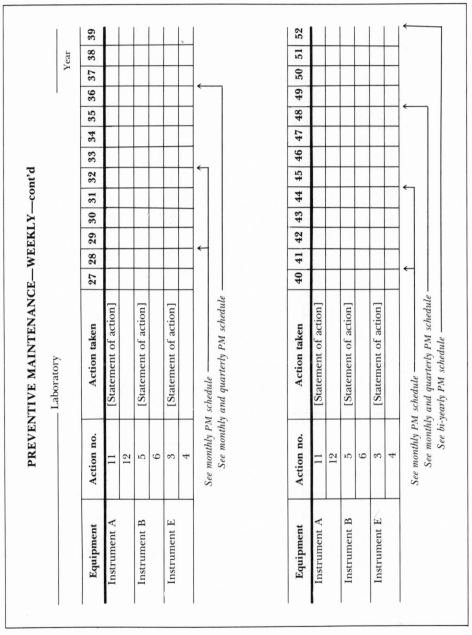

PREVENTIVE MAINTENANCE—WEEKLY—cont'd

———————— Laboratory

Year ————————

Equipment	Action no.	Action taken	27	28	29	30	31	32	33	34	35	36	37	38	39
Instrument A	11	[Statement of action]													
	12														
Instrument B	5	[Statement of action]													
	6														
Instrument E	3	[Statement of action]													
	4														

See monthly PM schedule ————————
See monthly and quarterly PM schedule ————————

Equipment	Action no.	Action taken	40	41	42	43	44	45	46	47	48	49	50	51	52
Instrument A	11	[Statement of action]													
	12														
Instrument B	5	[Statement of action]													
	6														
Instrument E	3	[Statement of action]													
	4														

See monthly PM schedule ————————
See monthly and quarterly PM schedule ————————
See bi-yearly PM schedule ————————

PREVENTIVE MAINTENANCE—MONTHLY

Laboratory _____   Year _____

Equipment	Action no.	Action taken	1	2	3	4	5	6	7	8	9	10	11	12
Instrument A	13	[Statement of action]												
	14													
Instrument G	4	[Statement of action]												
	5													
Instrument E	5	[Statement of action]												
	6													

See quarterly PM schedule →
See quarterly and bi-yearly PM schedule →
See quarterly, bi-yearly and yearly PM schedule →

PREVENTIVE MAINTENANCE—QUARTERLY

Equipment	Action no.	Action taken	1	2	3	4
Instrument C	3	[Statement of action]				
	4					
	5					
	6					
Instrument H	4	[Statement of action]				
	5					
	6					
	7					
	8					
	9					
	10					
	11					
	12					

See bi-yearly PM schedule →
See bi-yearly and yearly PM schedule →

PREVENTIVE MAINTENANCE—BI-YEARLY

Laboratory _____   Year _____

Equipment	Action no.	Action taken	1	2
Instrument A	15	[Statement of action]		
	16			
Instrument D	4	[Statement of action]		
	5			
Instrument C	7	[Statement of action]		
	8			
	9			

See yearly PM schedule

PREVENTIVE MAINTENANCE—YEARLY

Equipment	Action no.	Action taken
Instrument F	3	[Statement of action]
	4	
Instrument D	6	[Statement of action]
	7	
Instrument I	1	[Statement of action]
	2	
Instrument J	1	[Statement of action]
	2	

PREVENTIVE MAINTENANCE ACTION METHODS

_____ Laboratory

Equipment	Action no.	Description of action methods
Instrument A	1	[Concise instructions for performing
	2	this action method]
	3	
	4	
	5	
	6	
	7	
	8	
	9	
	10	
	11	
	12	
	13	
	14	
	15	
	16	
Instrument B	1	[Concise instructions for performing
	2	this action method]
	3	
	4	
	5	
	6	
Instrument C	1	[Concise instructions for performing
	2	this action method]
	3	
	4	
	5	
	6	
	7	
	8	
	9	

Continued.

PREVENTIVE MAINTENANCE ACTION METHODS–cont'd

_____ Laboratory

Equipment	Action no,	Description of action methods
Instrument D	1	[Concise instructions for performing
	2	this action method]
	3	
	4	
	5	
	6	
	7	
Instrument E	1	[Concise instructions for performing
	2	this action method]
	3	
	4	
	5	
	6	
Instrument F	1	[Concise instructions for performing
	2	this action method]
	3	
	4	
Instrument G	1	[Concise instructions for performing
	2	this action method]
	3	
	4	
	5	
Instrument H	1	[Concise instructions for performing
	2	this action method]
	3	
	4	
	5	
	6	
	7	
	8	
	9	
	10	
	11	
	12	
Instrument I	1	[Concise instructions for performing
	2	this action method]
Instrument J	1	[Concise instructions for performing
	2	this action method]

EQUIPMENT PERFORMANCE—6 MONTH SUMMARY

_____ Laboratory

_____
Year

Equipment	Performance
Instrument A	
Instrument B	
Instrument C	
Instrument D	
Instrument E	
Instrument F	
Instrument G	
Instrument H	
Instrument I	
Instrument J	

Denote performance by: 1 = No Problems; 2 = Few Problems (explain);
3 = Frequent Problems (explain).

EQUIPMENT PERFORMANCE—12 MONTH SUMMARY

_____ Laboratory

_____
Year

Equipment	Performance
Instrument A	
Instrument B	
Instrument C	
Instrument D	
Instrument E	
Instrument F	
Instrument G	
Instrument H	
Instrument I	
Instrument J	

Denote performance by: 1 = No Problems; 2 = Few Problems (explain);
3 = Frequent Problems (explain).

Department of Laboratories

WORKLOAD AND REVENUE FORECAST FORM

For fiscal year ending _____ _____ Laboratory

Test	In-patients				Out-patients				Other				Total no.	Total amt. ($)
	1st qtr.	2nd qtr.	3rd qtr.	4th qtr.	1st qtr.	2nd qtr.	3rd qtr.	4th qtr.	1st qtr.	2nd qtr.	3rd qtr.	4th qtr.		

Department of Laboratories

BUDGET FORM

For fiscal year ending ———————————   ——————————— Laboratory

Item	1st qtr. ($)	2nd qtr. ($)	3rd qtr. ($)	4th qtr. ($)	Total ($)
Salaries, exempt					
Salaries, nonexempt					
Supplies					
Equipment, purchase					
Equipment, lease					
Equipment, rental					
Equipment, maint.					
Ref. lab. fees					
Cont. ed. & travel					
Subscript. & dues					
R & D					
Depreciation					
Telephone					
Housekeeping					
Maint. (hosp.)					
Electricity					
Gen. hosp. admin.					
Taxes, payroll					
Taxes, sales					
Insur. gen. lab.					
Insur. work. comp.					
Insur. gr. health					
Insur. disability					
Insur. other					
Miscellaneous					
TOTAL					

Department of Laboratories

WORKLOAD AND REVENUE REPORT FORM

For period ending _____   Laboratory _____

Tests	Current quarter							Year-to-date						
	Forecast		Actual		Deviation			Forecast		Actual		Deviation	
	No.	Amt. ($)	No.	Amt. ($)	No.	Amt. ($)		No.	Amt. ($)	No.	Amt. ($)	No.	Amt. ($)

Department of Laboratories

BUDGET REPORT FORM

For period ending _____   _____ Laboratory

Item	Current quarter (in dollars)			Year-to-date (in dollars)		
	Budget	Actual	Deviation	Budget	Actual	Deviation
Salaries, exempt						
Salaries, nonexempt						
Supplies						
Equipment, purchase						
Equipment, lease						
Equipment, rental						
Equipment, maint.						
Ref. lab. fees						
Cont. ed. & travel						
Subscript. & dues						
R & D						
Depreciation						
Telephone						
Housekeeping						
Maint. (hosp.)						
Electricity						
Gen. hosp. admin.						
Taxes, payroll						
Taxes, sales						
Insur., gen. liab.						
Insur., work. comp.						
Insur., gr. health						
Insur., disability						
Insur., other						
Miscellaneous						
TOTAL						

Department of Laboratories

CAPITAL EQUIPMENT REQUEST FORM

_____ Laboratory

For fiscal year ending _____   _____ , Supervisor

Item _____

Brief description _____

_____

_____

_____

Source(s) _____

_____

Price _____

Return on investment _____

Justification   Priorities

☐ Replacement   ☐ Essential

☐ Increased volume   ☐ Necessary

☐ Cost reduction   ☐ Economically desirable

☐ New and/or improved procedure(s)   ☐ Other

_____

Date

_____

Signature

INVENTORY CARD

Item					Unit				
Minimum	**Maximum**		**Price**		**Catalogue number and information**				
Date	**P.O. no.**	**In**	**Out**	**Bal.**	**Date**	**P.O. no.**	**In**	**Out**	**Bal.**

Item—exact name as stated by the manufacturer and/or supplier.
Unit—smallest quantity that is customarily packaged and sold.
Price—price per unit.
Catalogue number and information—manufacturer and/or supplier and catalogue number.
Date—day, month, and year item is used and/or replenished.
P.O. no.—purchase order number.
In—number of units of item replenished.
Out—number of units of item issued.
Bal.—current number of units of item on hand.

FINANCIAL

SUMMATION   Summation is another way of expressing addition. It is symbolized by the Greek letter Σ (sigma), and most often used as a shorthand device for the addition of a series of numbers or terms. For example, the sum S of a series of numbers from 1 to 10 is

$$S = 1 + 2 + 3 + 4 + 5 + 6 + 7 + 8 + 9 + 10 = 55$$

and can be expressed as

$$\sum_{i=1}^{i=10} N_i = 55$$

where i represents a continuous series of N.

If we have a series of terms to add, the sum S is

$$S = \left(\frac{7}{128} \times 6\right) + \left(\frac{7}{128} \times 7\right) + \left(\frac{7}{128} \times 8\right) + \left(\frac{7}{128} \times 9\right)$$

We can represent the same required additions by simply writing

$$S = \sum_{i=6}^{i=9} \frac{7}{128} N_i$$

and further simplify the expression by factoring the coefficient to yield

$$S = \frac{7}{128} \sum_{i=6}^{i=9} N_i$$

If the coefficients are not equal to each other, then the summation, which assumes a more general form, becomes

$$S = \sum_{i=1}^{i=n} c_i N_i$$

WEIGHTED AVERAGE

The concept of weighted average is useful especially for planning and estimating purposes. Essentially, it incorporates the degree of importance to each of those elements to be averaged. Such assignment of importance is called weighting, hence the weighted average.

Example 1

A physician is requesting price quotations for catecholamines, urinalysis, and VMA. He estimates that he would be submitting ten specimens for catecholamines, twenty-five for urinalysis, and fifteen for VMA each month. The unit prices given to the physician are $30.00, $5.00 and $20.00 for catecholamines, urinalysis, and VMA, respectively.

The unadjusted average price would be $18.33 per test. However, such unadjusted average is not a useful parameter because the test volume and the prices are unevenly distributed. To account for the uneven distribution, we should weight the average as follows:

A_w = Weighted average price =

$$\frac{10}{50}(\$30.00) + \frac{25}{50}(\$5.00) + \frac{15}{50}(\$20.00) = \$14.50 \text{ per test}$$

The weighting factor becomes the ratio of the number of each given test to the total number of tests.

As long as the physician continues to submit specimens in approximately the same ratio, the total estimated laboratory revenue generated by him is simply the product of the total number of specimens and the weighted average price. The concept of weighted average can be used in more precise manners as illustrated by the following case.

191

Example 2   A hospital laboratory is contemplating the purchase of a $4,000 densitometer. The hospital has two methods to finance the purchase. The first involves a loan of $4,000 at 7.9 percent interest. The second is a combination package: a special loan of $2,000 at 9 percent interest, $1,000 from retained earnings requiring a 5 percent return, and $1,000 at 8 percent interest from the hospital capital pool. Which method of finance would be preferred?

The weighted average cost of capital for the combination package method is

$$A_w = \frac{2,000}{4,000}(9.00\%) + \frac{1,000}{4,000}(5.00\%) + \frac{1,000}{4,000}(8.00\%) = 7.75\%$$

Therefore, the combination package method is preferred.

The weighted average concept becomes even more useful when there are many widely distributed elements to be averaged. In general, the weighted average (A_w) is expressed as follows:

$$A_w = \frac{x_1}{N}(P_1) + \frac{x_2}{N}(P_2) + \frac{x_3}{N}(P_3) + \cdots$$

where P represents the entity to be weighted, x the weight element in P, and N the sum of all the x's.

TABLE C-1

The compound sum of $1.00 for n periods

n	1%	2%	3%	4%	5%	6%	7%	8%	9%	10%
1	1.010	1.020	1.030	1.040	1.050	1.060	1.070	1.080	1.090	1.100
2	1.020	1.040	1.061	1.082	1.103	1.124	1.145	1.166	1.188	1.210
3	1.030	1.061	1.093	1.125	1.158	1.191	1.225	1.260	1.295	1.331
4	1.041	1.082	1.126	1.170	1.216	1.262	1.311	1.360	1.412	1.464
5	1.051	1.104	1.159	1.217	1.276	1.338	1.403	1.469	1.539	1.611
6	1.062	1.126	1.194	1.265	1.340	1.419	1.501	1.587	1.677	1.772
7	1.072	1.149	1.230	1.316	1.407	1.504	1.606	1.714	1.828	1.949
8	1.083	1.172	1.267	1.369	1.477	1.594	1.718	1.851	1.993	2.144
9	1.094	1.195	1.305	1.423	1.551	1.689	1.838	1.999	2.172	2.358
10	1.105	1.219	1.344	1.480	1.629	1.791	1.967	2.159	2.367	2.594
11	1.116	1.243	1.384	1.539	1.710	1.898	2.105	2.332	2.580	2.853
12	1.127	1.268	1.426	1.601	1.796	2.012	2.252	2.518	2.813	3.138
13	1.138	1.294	1.469	1.665	1.886	2.133	2.410	2.720	3.066	3.452
14	1.149	1.319	1.513	1.732	1.980	2.261	2.579	2.937	3.342	3.797
15	1.161	1.346	1.558	1.801	2.079	2.397	2.759	3.172	3.642	4.177
16	1.173	1.373	1.605	1.873	2.183	2.540	2.952	3.426	3.970	4.595
17	1.184	1.400	1.653	1.948	2.292	2.693	3.159	3.700	4.328	5.054
18	1.196	1.428	1.702	2.026	2.407	2.854	3.380	3.996	4.717	5.560
19	1.208	1.457	1.754	2.107	2.527	3.026	3.617	4.316	5.142	6.116
20	1.220	1.486	1.806	2.191	2.653	3.207	3.870	4.661	5.604	6.727
21	1.232	1.516	1.860	2.279	2.786	3.400	4.141	5.034	6.109	7.400
22	1.245	1.546	1.916	2.370	2.925	3.604	4.430	5.437	6.659	8.140
23	1.257	1.577	1.974	2.465	3.072	3.820	4.741	5.871	7.258	8.954
24	1.270	1.608	2.033	2.563	3.225	4.049	5.072	6.341	7.911	9.850
25	1.282	1.641	2.094	2.666	3.386	4.292	5.427	6.848	8.623	10.83
26	1.295	1.673	2.157	2.772	3.556	4.549	5.807	7.396	9.399	11.92
27	1.308	1.707	2.221	2.883	3.733	4.822	6.214	7.988	10.25	13.11
28	1.321	1.741	2.288	2.999	3.920	4.112	6.649	8.627	11.17	14.42
29	1.335	1.776	2.357	3.119	4.116	5.418	7.114	9.317	12.17	15.86
30	1.348	1.811	2.427	3.243	4.322	5.743	7.612	10.06	13.27	17.45

Continued.

TABLE C-1
The compound sum of $1.00 for n periods—cont'd

n	11%	12%	13%	14%	15%	16%	17%	18%	19%	20%
1	1.110	1.120	1.130	1.140	1.150	1.160	1.170	1.180	1.190	1.200
2	1.232	1.254	1.277	1.300	1.323	1.346	1.369	1.392	1.416	1.440
3	1.368	1.405	1.443	1.482	1.521	1.561	1.602	1.643	1.685	1.728
4	1.518	1.574	1.630	1.689	1.749	1.811	1.874	1.939	2.005	2.074
5	1.685	1.762	1.842	1.925	2.011	2.100	2.192	2.288	2.386	2.488
6	1.870	1.974	2.082	2.195	2.313	2.436	2.565	2.700	2.840	2.986
7	2.076	2.211	2.353	2.502	2.660	2.826	3.001	3.185	3.379	3.583
8	2.305	2.476	2.658	2.853	3.059	3.278	3.511	3.759	4.021	4.300
9	2.558	2.773	3.004	3.252	3.518	3.803	4.108	4.435	4.785	5.160
10	2.839	3.106	3.395	3.707	4.046	4.411	4.807	5.234	5.695	6.192
11	3.152	3.479	3.836	4.226	4.652	5.117	5.624	6.176	6.777	7.430
12	3.498	3.896	4.335	4.818	5.350	5.936	6.580	7.288	8.064	8.916
13	3.883	4.363	4.898	5.492	6.153	6.886	7.699	8.600	9.596	10.70
14	4.310	4.887	5.535	6.261	7.076	7.988	9.007	10.15	11.42	12.84
15	4.785	5.474	6.254	7.138	8.137	9.266	10.54	11.97	13.59	15.41
16	5.311	6.130	7.067	8.137	9.358	10.75	12.33	14.13	16.17	18.49
17	5.895	6.866	7.986	9.276	10.76	12.47	14.43	16.67	19.24	22.19
18	6.544	7.690	9.024	10.58	12.38	14.46	16.88	19.67	22.90	26.62
19	7.263	8.613	10.20	12.06	14.23	16.78	19.75	23.21	27.25	31.95
20	8.062	9.646	11.52	13.74	16.37	19.46	23.11	27.39	32.43	38.34
21	8.949	10.80	13.02	15.67	18.82	22.57	27.03	32.32	38.59	46.01
22	9.934	12.10	14.71	17.86	21.64	26.19	31.63	38.14	45.92	55.21
23	11.03	13.55	16.63	20.36	24.89	30.38	37.01	45.01	54.65	56.25
24	12.24	15.18	18.79	23.21	28.63	35.24	43.30	53.11	65.03	79.50
25	13.59	17.00	21.23	26.46	32.92	40.87	50.66	62.67	77.39	95.40
26	15.08	19.04	23.99	30.17	37.86	47.41	59.27	73.95	92.09	114.5
27	16.74	21.32	27.11	34.39	43.54	55.00	69.35	87.26	109.6	137.4
28	18.58	23.88	30.63	39.20	50.07	63.80	81.13	103.0	130.4	164.8
29	20.62	26.75	34.62	44.69	57.58	74.01	94.93	121.5	155.2	197.8
30	22.89	29.96	39.12	50.95	66.21	85.85	111.1	143.4	184.7	237.4

TABLE C-1
The compound sum of $1.00 for n periods—cont'd

n	21%	22%	23%	24%	25%	26%	27%	28%	29%	30%
1	1.210	1.220	1.230	1.240	1.250	1.260	1.270	1.280	1.290	1.300
2	1.464	1.488	1.513	1.538	1.563	1.588	1.613	1.638	1.664	1.690
3	1.772	1.816	1.861	1.907	1.953	2.000	2.048	2.097	2.147	2.856
4	2.144	2.215	2.289	2.364	2.441	2.520	2.601	2.684	2.769	3.713
5	2.594	2.703	2.815	2.932	3.052	3.176	3.304	3.436	3.572	4.827
6	3.138	3.297	3.463	3.635	3.815	4.002	4.196	4.398	4.608	6.275
7	3.797	4.023	4.259	4.508	4.768	5.042	5.329	5.629	5.945	8.157
8	4.595	4.908	5.239	5.590	5.960	6.353	6.768	7.206	7.669	10.60
9	5.560	5.987	6.444	6.931	7.451	8.005	8.595	9.223	9.893	13.79
10	6.727	7.305	7.926	8.594	9.313	10.09	10.92	11.81	12.76	17.92
11	8.140	8.912	9.749	10.66	11.64	12.71	13.86	15.11	16.46	23.30
12	9.850	10.87	11.99	13.21	14.55	16.01	17.61	19.34	21.24	30.29
13	11.92	13.26	14.75	16.39	18.19	20.18	22.36	24.76	27.39	39.37
14	14.42	16.18	18.14	20.32	22.74	25.42	28.40	31.69	35.34	51.19
15	17.45	19.74	22.31	25.20	28.42	32.03	36.06	40.56	45.59	66.54
16	21.11	24.09	27.45	31.24	35.53	40.36	45.80	51.92	58.81	86.50
17	25.55	29.38	33.76	38.74	44.41	50.85	58.17	66.46	75.86	112.5
18	30.91	35.85	41.52	48.04	55.51	64.07	73.87	85.07	97.86	146.2
19	37.40	43.74	51.07	59.57	69.39	80.73	93.81	108.9	126.2	190.0
20	45.26	53.36	62.82	73.86	86.74	101.7	119.1	139.4	162.9	247.1
21	54.76	65.10	77.27	91.59	108.4	128.2	151.3	178.4	210.1	321.2
22	66.26	79.42	95.04	113.6	135.5	161.5	192.2	228.4	271.0	417.5
23	80.18	96.89	116.9	140.8	169.4	203.5	244.1	292.3	349.6	542.8
24	97.02	118.2	143.8	174.6	211.8	256.4	309.9	374.1	451.0	705.6
25	117.4	144.2	176.9	216.5	264.7	323.0	393.6	478.9	581.8	917.3
26	142.0	175.9	217.5	268.5	330.9	407.0	499.9	613.0	750.5	1193
27	171.9	214.6	267.6	333.0	413.6	512.9	634.6	784.6	968.1	1550
28	208.0	261.9	329.1	412.9	517.0	646.2	806.3	1004	1249	2015
29	251.6	319.5	404.8	512.0	646.2	814.2	1024	1286	1611	2620
30	304.5	389.8	497.9	634.8	807.8	1026	1301	1646	2078	3406

TABLE C-2
The present value of $1.00 for n periods

n	1%	2%	3%	4%	5%	6%	7%	8%	9%	10%
1	.990	.980	.971	.962	.952	.943	.935	.926	.917	.909
2	.980	.961	.943	.925	.907	.890	.873	.857	.842	.826
3	.971	.942	.915	.889	.864	.840	.816	.794	.772	.751
4	.961	.924	.888	.855	.823	.792	.763	.735	.708	.683
5	.951	.906	.863	.822	.784	.747	.713	.681	.650	.621
6	.942	.888	.837	.790	.746	.705	.666	.630	.596	.564
7	.933	.871	.813	.760	.711	.665	.623	.583	.547	.513
8	.923	.853	.789	.731	.677	.627	.582	.540	.502	.467
9	.914	.837	.766	.703	.645	.592	.544	.500	.460	.424
10	.905	.820	.744	.676	.614	.558	.508	.463	.422	.386
11	.896	.804	.722	.650	.585	.527	.475	.429	.388	.350
12	.887	.788	.701	.625	.557	.497	.444	.397	.356	.319
13	.879	.773	.681	.601	.530	.469	.415	.368	.326	.290
14	.870	.758	.661	.577	.505	.442	.388	.340	.299	.263
15	.861	.743	.642	.555	.481	.417	.362	.315	.275	.239
16	.853	.728	.623	.534	.458	.394	.339	.292	.252	.218
17	.844	.714	.605	.513	.436	.371	.317	.270	.231	.198
18	.836	.700	.587	.494	.416	.350	.296	.250	.212	.180
19	.828	.684	.570	.475	.396	.331	.277	.232	.194	.164
20	.820	.673	.554	.456	.377	.312	.258	.215	.178	.149
21	.811	.660	.538	.439	.359	.294	.242	.199	.164	.135
22	.803	.647	.522	.422	.342	.278	.226	.184	.150	.123
23	.795	.634	.507	.406	.326	.262	.211	.170	.138	.112
24	.788	.622	.492	.390	.310	.247	.197	.158	.126	.102
25	.780	.610	.478	.375	.295	.233	.184	.146	.116	.092
26	.772	.598	.464	.361	.281	.220	.172	.135	.106	.084
27	.764	.586	.450	.347	.268	.207	.161	.125	.098	.076
28	.757	.574	.437	.333	.255	.196	.150	.116	.090	.069
29	.749	.563	.424	.320	.243	.185	.141	.107	.082	.063
30	.742	.552	.412	.308	.231	.174	.131	.099	.075	.057

TABLE C-2

The present values of $1.00 for n periods—cont'd

n	11%	12%	13%	14%	15%	16%	17%	18%	19%	20%
1	.901	.893	.885	.877	.870	.862	.855	.847	.840	.833
2	.812	.797	.783	.769	.756	.743	.731	.718	.706	.694
3	.731	.712	.693	.675	.658	.641	.624	.609	.593	.579
4	.659	.636	.613	.592	.572	.552	.534	.516	.499	.482
5	.593	.567	.543	.519	.497	.476	.456	.437	.419	.402
6	.535	.507	.480	.456	.432	.410	.390	.370	.352	.335
7	.482	.453	.425	.400	.376	.354	.333	.314	.296	.279
8	.434	.404	.376	.351	.327	.305	.285	.266	.249	.233
9	.391	.361	.333	.308	.284	.263	.243	.225	.209	.194
10	.352	.322	.295	.270	.247	.227	.208	.191	.176	.162
11	.317	.287	.261	.237	.215	.195	.178	.162	.148	.135
12	.286	.257	.231	.208	.187	.168	.152	.137	.124	.112
13	.258	.229	.204	.182	.163	.145	.130	.116	.104	.093
14	.232	.205	.181	.160	.141	.125	.111	.099	.088	.078
15	.209	.183	.160	.140	.123	.108	.095	.084	.074	.065
16	.188	.163	.141	.123	.107	.093	.081	.071	.062	.054
17	.170	.146	.125	.108	.093	.080	.069	.060	.052	.045
18	.153	.130	.111	.095	.081	.069	.059	.051	.044	.038
19	.138	.116	.098	.083	.070	.058	.051	.043	.037	.031
20	.124	.104	.087	.073	.061	.050	.043	.037	.031	.028
21	.112	.093	.077	.064	.053	.043	.037	.031	.026	.022
22	.101	.083	.068	.056	.046	.037	.032	.026	.022	.018
23	.091	.074	.060	.049	.040	.032	.027	.022	.018	.015
24	.082	.066	.053	.043	.035	.028	.023	.019	.015	.013
25	.074	.059	.047	.038	.030	.024	.020	.016	.013	.010
26	.066	.053	.042	.033	.026	.021	.017	.014	.011	.009
27	.060	.047	.037	.029	.023	.018	.014	.012	.009	.007
28	.054	.042	.033	.026	.020	.015	.012	.010	.008	.006
29	.048	.037	.029	.022	.017	.013	.011	.008	.006	.005
30	.044	.033	.026	.020	.015	.011	.009	.007	.005	.004

Continued.

TABLE C-2

The present values of $1.00 for n periods—cont'd

n	21%	22%	23%	24%	25%	26%	27%	28%	29%	30%
1	.826	.820	.813	.806	.800	.794	.787	.781	.775	.769
2	.683	.672	.661	.650	.640	.630	.620	.610	.601	.592
3	.564	.551	.537	.524	.512	.500	.488	.477	.466	.455
4	.467	.451	.437	.423	.410	.397	.384	.373	.361	.350
5	.386	.370	.355	.341	.328	.315	.303	.291	.280	.269
6	.319	.303	.289	.275	.262	.250	.238	.227	.217	.207
7	.263	.249	.235	.222	.210	.198	.188	.178	.168	.159
8	.218	.204	.191	.179	.168	.157	.148	.139	.130	.123
9	.180	.167	.155	.144	.134	.125	.116	.108	.101	.094
10	.149	.137	.126	.116	.107	.099	.092	.085	.078	.073
11	.123	.112	.103	.094	.086	.079	.072	.066	.061	.056
12	.102	.092	.083	.076	.069	.062	.057	.052	.047	.043
13	.084	.075	.068	.061	.055	.050	.045	.040	.037	.033
14	.069	.062	.055	.049	.044	.039	.035	.032	.028	.025
15	.057	.051	.045	.040	.035	.031	.028	.025	.022	.020
16	.047	.042	.036	.032	.028	.025	.022	.019	.017	.015
17	.039	.034	.030	.026	.023	.020	.017	.015	.013	.012
18	.032	.028	.024	.021	.018	.016	.014	.012	.010	.009
19	.027	.023	.020	.017	.014	.012	.011	.009	.008	.007
20	.022	.019	.016	.014	.012	.010	.008	.007	.006	.005
21	.018	.015	.013	.011	.009	.008	.007	.006	.005	.004
22	.015	.013	.011	.009	.007	.006	.005	.004	.004	.003
23	.012	.010	.009	.007	.006	.005	.004	.003	.003	.002
24	.010	.008	.007	.006	.005	.004	.003	.003	.002	.002
25	.009	.007	.006	.005	.004	.003	.003	.002	.002	.001
26	.007	.006	.005	.004	.003	.002	.002	.002	.001	.001
27	.006	.005	.004	.003	.002	.002	.002	.001	.001	.001
28	.005	.004	.003	.002	.002	.002	.001	.001	.001	.001
29	.004	.003	.002	.002	.002	.001	.001	.001	.001	.000
30	.003	.003	.002	.002	.001	.001	.001	.001	.000	.000

Depreciation is the reduction of the value of an asset re- **DEPRECIATION**
sulting from usage, deterioration, consumption, or aging.
The usual methods for calculating depreciation are: (1)
straight line, (2) sum-of-years-digits, and (3) double declining balance. The latter two are also known as accelerated
depreciation methods.

Assume that a spectrophotometer purchased for $6,600
has an estimated useful life of ten years and a salvage value
of $600 at the end of the tenth year. The results of different
methods of its depreciation are listed below.

Comparison of depreciation methods

Year	Straight line	Sum-of-years-digits	Double declining balance
1	$600	$1,091	$1,320
2	600	982	1,056
3	600	873	845
4	600	764	676
5	600	655	541
6	600	545	432
7	600	436	346
8	600	327	277
9	600	218	221
10	600	109	177*
TOTAL	$6,000	$6,000	$5,891

*At the end of the tenth year there is a residual amount of $109 for the double declining balance method of accounting for depreciation.

The straight line depreciation method provides a uniform **Straight line**
depreciation charge each year as follows:

$$\text{Annual depreciation D} = \frac{(\text{Cost}) - (\text{salvage value})}{(\text{Years of useful life})}$$

For the spectrophotometer

$$\text{Annual depreciation D} = \frac{\$6,600 - \$600}{10} = \$600/\text{yr.}$$

Notice that the asset is depreciating at the constant rate
of 10% each year.

Sum-of-years-digits

With the sum-of-years-digits method, the sum (S) of the years is first determined

$$S = \frac{N(N + 1)}{2}$$

where N is the number of years of useful life.

In our example, we have

$$S = \frac{10(10 + 1)}{2} = 55$$

The depreciation, D_i, for the ith year is expressed by the following:

$$D_i = \frac{R}{S} (\text{Cost} - \text{salvage value})$$

where R stands for the number of remaining years. The depreciation for the spectrophotometer under this method then is shown at top of p. 201.

Notice that the depreciation rate is not constant, being more rapid in earlier years and slowing to less than that of the straight line method.

Double declining balance

The double declining balance method applies a constant yearly rate of depreciation, usually twice the straight line depreciation rate, to the undepreciated value of the asset. In this method, the undepreciated value is the full purchase price of the spectrophotometer, not the cost less salvage value. It can be calculated with the following expression:

$$D'_i = K (\text{purchase price} - \text{accumulated depreciation})$$

where D'_i represents the double declining balance depreciation for the ith year and K the constant depreciation rate. For our example, we have the tabulated calculations on the bottom of p. 201.

With this method, the asset is not fully depreciated at the end of its useful life. The residual, however, would be depreciated during the last year of the asset's useful life.

Sum-of-years-digits depreciation

Year	Depreciation
1	$\frac{10}{55} \times (6{,}600 - 600) = \$1{,}091$
2	$\frac{9}{55} \times (6{,}600 - 600) = \quad 982$
3	$\frac{8}{55} \times (6{,}600 - 600) = \quad 873$
4	$\frac{7}{55} \times (6{,}600 - 600) = \quad 764$
5	$\frac{6}{55} \times (6{,}600 - 600) = \quad 655$
6	$\frac{5}{55} \times (6{,}600 - 600) = \quad 545$
7	$\frac{4}{55} \times (6{,}600 - 600) = \quad 436$
8	$\frac{3}{55} \times (6{,}600 - 600) = \quad 327$
9	$\frac{2}{55} \times (6{,}600 - 600) = \quad 218$
10	$\frac{1}{55} \times (6{,}600 - 600) = \quad 109$

Double declining balance depreciation

Year	K		Purchase price		Accumulated depreciation		D'_i	Residual
1	0.2	×	(6,600	−	0)	=	1,320	
2	0.2	×	(6,600	−	1,320)	=	1,056	
3	0.2	×	(6,600	−	2,376)	=	845	
4	0.2	×	(6,600	−	3,221)	=	676	
5	0.2	×	(6,600	−	3,897)	=	541	
6	0.2	×	(6,600	−	4,439)	=	432	
7	0.2	×	(6,600	−	4,870)	=	346	
8	0.2	×	(6,600	−	5,216)	=	277	
9	0.2	×	(6,600	−	5,493)	=	221	
10	0.2	×	(6,600	−	5,714)	=	177	
TOTAL							$5,891	109

201

INDEX